Recovery from Addiction in Communal Living Settings

T0264739

Research on treatment outcome for addictive disorders indicates that a variety of interventions are effective. However, the progress clients make in treatment frequently is undermined by the lack of an alcohol and drug free living environment supporting sustained recovery. This book suggests that treatment providers have not paid sufficient attention to the social environments where clients live after residential treatment or while attending outpatient programs. It also describes the need for alcohol and drug free living environments.

We then review the history of communal living for recovering addicts and alcoholics and provide concrete examples of the Oxford House model, which is a widespread communal living option for over 10,000 recovering persons in the US. The structure and philosophy of Oxford Houses are presented along with recent outcome studies providing support for their effectiveness.

This book was published as a special issue in the *Journal of Groups in Addiction and Recovery*.

Leonard A. Jason is the Director of the Center for Community Research and a Professor of Psychology at DePaul University. His research interests include recovery homes and addiction, tobacco prevention interventions, and chronic fatigue syndrome.

Joseph R. Ferrari, Ph.D. is the Vincent Distinguished Professor of Psychology at DePaul University and his interests include; chronic procrastination, self-handicapping and attribution, attitude change and persuasion, community-based service-learning &and volunteerism, community Building and sense of community, recovery from addiction, and behavior analysis in the community.

Recovery from Addiction in Communal Living Settings

The Oxford House Model

Edited by

Leonard A. Jason and Joseph R. Ferrari

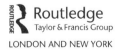

Routledge
Taylor & Francis Group

LONDON AND NEW YORK

Contents

CONTENTS

Oxford House Effects on the External Community

Introduction: Using the Oxford House Model to Examine 12-Step Recovery

This book has been organized to illustrate the contributions of Leonard Jason and Joseph Ferrari to our understanding of 12-step recovery as originally developed by Alcoholics Anonymous (AA). While research on AA has been limited by the role of anonymity in recovery, the willingness of the Oxford Houses to open their doors to academic research gives us an opportunity to see recovery from addiction in action. We observe that the 12 steps move the recovering addict from the internal changes that occur with abstinence and surrender (Steps One, Two and Three) to changes in the interpersonal realm (Steps Four, Five, Six, and Seven) that lead to changes in the recovering addicts' relationship with the community (Steps Eight, Nine, Ten, Eleven, and Twelve). I suggest that the book informs us about how groups of recovering addicts living together practice these 12 steps.

1. We admitted we were powerless over alcohol—that our lives had become unmanageable.

The first word of the first step, "we," may be the most important word of the 12 steps. The introductory chapter by Polcin emphasizes the significance of communal living as a support for recovery from addiction. The experience of living in a community of people working together toward a common purpose may be the first opportunity for the recovering addict to become part of a "we." Alcoholics refer to the "ism" of alcoholism as meaning "I sponsor myself" (otherwise interpreted humorously as incredibly short memory). The isolation involved in not being able to depend on other people for emotional support provides fertile ground for addiction. Ironically, then, the path to self-efficacy involves letting go of self-sufficiency. In this regard, the freedom that the Oxford Houses give to their residents to attend or not to attend formal 12-step meetings is paradoxical. According to the received wisdom of AA, any gathering of two or more alcoholics who come together to share their experience, strength, and hope about recovery from alcoholism constitutes a meeting of AA. Using this definition, the Oxford House model provides the opportunity to be in a 12-step meeting 24-7.

2. We came to believe that a Power greater than ourselves could restore us to sanity.

While many of us confuse this spiritual step with religion, for group therapists, the idea that a group can achieve goals working together that the individual would find impossible is second nature. Here again, the received wisdom of AA is helpful, instructing us that the alcoholic's first recognition of a Higher Power may come from the AA meeting itself. If we recognize addiction as a family disease, then the family that has been affected by addiction has been unable to offer its members the experience of a Higher Power that leads to sanity. The article by Groh et al. demonstrates the synergistic principle that many forces acting together produce a more useful product than any of these forces produce alone. Using the experience of belonging to a 12-step group or of living in an Oxford House to come to believe that help is available outside of oneself may lead to a dramatic shift in the addict's relationship with the world outside.

3. We made a decision to turn our will and our lives over to the care of God as we understood Him.

The article by Ferrari et al. provides an excellent illustration of the utility of the Oxford House studies in understanding how 12-step recovery intersects with our commonplace understanding of impulse control. When we are studying the individual, we may focus on self-regulation and self-efficacy, as if the individual functions in social isolation, instead of drawing on interpersonal support to maintain emotional and psychological homeostasis. Indeed, one of the strengths of community psychology is its examination of the social forces that shape individual behavior. Addicts recovering using the 12-steps explicitly let go of self-will and surrender to being regulated by their recovering community, which becomes a primary representation of their Higher Power. The Oxford House residents in these studies, therefore, have all elected to use the Oxford House as an integral part of their Higher Power, to which they can turn over their impulses to use alcohol and drugs, thereby freeing up their limited intrapsychic resources to accomplish goals other than "white-knuckle" abstinence.

4. We made a searching and fearless moral inventory of ourselves.

The article by Mathis et al. amplifies the experience of hope in terms of agency, goals, and pathways. These concepts create a bridge between the surrender in Step Three and the beginning of an examination of oneself in Step Four. As the recovering addict in an Oxford House uses the agency that is available in a power outside of himself or herself, as do the other Oxford House residents, goals and pathways become available through the process of engaging in intimate interpersonal contact. The capacity to measure the attitudes and beliefs that characterize addiction and recovery moves us much closer to understanding the active ingredients of the 12-step programs.

5. We admitted to God, to ourselves and to another human being the exact nature of our wrongs.

The ability to be honest and transparent in one's interactions with others is a central value in recovery. The article by Groh et al. on social desirability sheds light on the challenges that the recovering addict faces in becoming rigorously honest. On the one hand, the impulse for social desirability may provide significant motivation for prosocial behavior, as described in a later article by Viola et al. On the other hand, wishing to be seen as desirable instead of acting in a manner conducive to attachment may lead to relapse as the distance between what is real and what is pretense becomes wider.

6. We were entirely ready to have God remove all these defects of character.

As the recovering addict becomes open to hope and the wish for social connection is rejuvenated, the addict may have the first experience of a psychological sense of community (PSOC) as described by Graham et al. If we understand addiction as a disease of isolation, then one primary "defect of character" may be the absence of this psychological sense of community. The ability to study the development of PSOC as a function of joining a community such as the Oxford House opens the possibility of understanding the broader PSOC that becomes available in the larger community of 12-step fellowships.

7. We humbly asked Him to remove our shortcomings.

Many of us locate in our children different visions and hopes for our future, and in this way, our children become part of a power outside of ourselves that may lead us to make decisions that delay immediate impulses in favor of building the structures that will support us in the future. That Ortiz et al. initiate an examination of the impact of children in Oxford Houses reminds us that many children grow up in families with addiction. Some of these children suffer permanent injury from this experience; some of these children may be fortunate enough to have one or both parents engaged in a process of recovery, thus providing a model for a way out of the insanity. The results of this preliminary study suggest support for a traditional piece of folk wisdom from AA: sometimes recovery involves contrary action, which is action that is the opposite of what one has been programmed to do as a practicing addict. If the role of men as practicing addicts frequently leads to abandonment of the family, and the role of women as practicing addicts frequently involves the experience of resenting having to take care of children, we may not be surprised that recovering addicts in the Oxford House model find support in moving out of their traditional, dysfunctional roles.

8. We made a list of all persons we had harmed and became willing to make amends to them all.

This step constitutes an acknowledgement on the addict's part that the disease of addiction, consistent with the unmanageability admitted to in Step One, has caused harm to self and others. One of the more measurable forms of harm may be the criminal and violent behavior often associated with addiction. While making amends is often understood as undoing the harmful behavior, a more immediate and practicable form of making amends may be simply abstaining from criminal and violent behavior. The article by Aase et al. addresses the issue directly and demonstrates that participation in the Oxford House model leads to changes in behavior, with decreased antisocial and increased prosocial behavior consistent with the process of making amends.

9. Made direct amends to such people wherever possible, except when to do so would injure them or others.

Just as the willingness to make amends for harms suffered in the past entails abstaining from criminal and violent behavior, so making direct amends entails joining the community in making productive contributions. Belyaev-Glantsman et al. provide convincing data that participation in the Oxford House model, and thus in 12-step recovery, correlates well with a return of the recovering addicts to gainful employment. Not unexpectedly, their progress in becoming employed improves with the duration of their recovery and is also limited by factors that affect the general population.

10. We continued to take personal inventory, and when we were wrong promptly admitted it.

11. Sought through prayer and meditation to improve our conscious contact with God, as we understood Him, praying only for knowledge of His will for us and the power to carry that out.

As the recovering addicts become part of the larger community in which the Oxford Houses are located, they are able to participate and contribute to the life of these communities. This process of reattachment requires two related capacities: continued self-examination accomplished with an openness to support from others and willingness to admit the inevitable mistakes that are part of being human and imperfect. If we understand meditation as the capacity to pay attention and listen to how we are responding to the larger world around us and prayer as the capacity to communicate our needs to this larger world that supports us, then the recovering addict's use of prayer and meditation to maintain a relationship with the larger community becomes comprehensible. The study of neighborhood environments of mutual-help recovery houses by Ferrari et al. represents a classic social and community psychology examination of the impact of a group of recovering addicts on their community and the impact of the community on the recovering addicts.

12. Having had a spiritual awakening as the result of these steps, we tried to carry this message to alcoholics and to practice these principles in all our affairs.

The final step of the 12 steps is often misinterpreted as guided by evangelical motives. While recovery from addiction may be experienced as a conversion from the culture of intoxication to a culture of sobriety, the motive of the recovering addict in "carrying the message" is entirely selfish: the maintenance of one's own sobriety. Again, the received wisdom of AA is that "in order to get it, you have to give it away." Perhaps not coincidentally, the article by Viola et al. on measuring helping behaviors in the Oxford Houses was the first article received by this journal, the article that inspired this book. It includes two studies on helping behaviors that illuminate the core features of how mutual support operates for the benefit of the addict who is helping and the addict who is helped. The results offer insight into the utility of sponsorship, a central mechanism of practicing Steps Two and Three. Recovering addicts are advised to find someone in their meetings who has what they want and to ask how they got it. The person who is asked for help may assume the role of sponsor, in doing so practicing the Twelfth Step.

We are grateful for the willingness of co-editors Leonard Jason and Joseph Ferrari, both for their commitment and sensitivity in organizing this book and for their genius and passion in creatively using the tools of social and community psychology to advance our understanding of the complex process of recovery from addiction. We hope that in your reading of the chapters that follow, you will find inspiration and increased recognition of the opportunities for research and clinical application of the principles of recovery from addiction in many different areas, including the internal life of the addict, the effects of recovery in the interpersonal realm, and the effects of recovery on the external community. If you can appreciate the breadth of what these authors are investigating, we suggest that "you will be amazed before you are half-way through."

Jeffrey D. Roth MD, FASAM

Communal-Living Settings for Adults Recovering from Substance Abuse

DOUGLAS L. POLCIN, EdD

Alcohol Research Group, Public Health Institute, Emeryville, California

Research on treatment outcome for addictive disorders indicates that a variety of interventions are effective. However, the progress clients make in treatment frequently is undermined by the lack of an alcohol- and drug-free living environment supporting sustained recovery. This introduction to a special edition on Oxford Houses suggests that treatment providers have not paid sufficient attention to the social environments where clients live after residential treatment or while attending outpatient programs. The article begins with a description of the need for alcohol- and drug-free living environments. The history of communal living for recovering addicts and alcoholics is then reviewed and the Oxford House model emphasized as a recent and widespread communal-living option for recovering persons. The structure and philosophy of Oxford Houses are presented along with recent outcome studies providing support for their effectiveness. Three different perspectives are presented as ways of conceptualizing how residents in Oxford Houses benefit: social context theory, self-governance or self-care, and peer affiliation or identification.

There is growing consensus in the addiction treatment field that a variety of interventions appear to be effective (National Institute on Drug Abuse [NIDA], 1999). Reviews showed that addiction treatment results in substantial decreases in substance use and improvements in related problem areas, such as family relationships, legal problems, medical status, psychiatric symptoms, and employment. Reviews of cost-benefit studies suggest taxpayers save up to $12 for every $1 spent on adult treatment for addiction (NIDA, 1999), primarily through reductions in criminal justice and healthcare expenses. The types of services included in these reviews encompass the entire spectrum of inpatient, outpatient, and methadone treatment.

Despite gains made as a result of treatment, at some point many clients experience episodes of relapse. Some clients require multiple admissions to treatment programs to sustain sobriety (NIDA, 1999). Maintaining abstinence from alcohol and drugs after completion of residential treatment or during outpatient treatment appears to be most challenging for clients who do not have stable living environments (Hitchcock, Stainback, & Roque, 1995; Milby, Schumacher, Wallace, Feedman, & Vuchinich, 1996) or social support systems that encourage abstinence (Moos & Moos, 2006).

Over the past 20 years the high cost of housing (especially in urban areas) was a major obstacle to creating stable living environments for persons in recovery. For example, a frequent complaint by residential treatment providers is the lack of affordable housing for clients who leave their facilities. When clients are released from residential programs into economically deprived neighborhoods that do not actively support abstinence, the recovery they established in treatment may be lost. Outpatient providers face a similar dilemma. Even if clients are engaged in outpatient treatment, motivated for change, and making improvements, their progress may be mitigated if they reside in a destructive living environment that triggers relapse (Polcin, Galloway, Taylor, & Benowitz-Fredericks, 2004).

Furthermore, individuals beyond persons in treatment may be impacted by the lack of alcohol- and drug-free living environments. For example, criminal justice offenders with a history of addiction problems released on parole rarely access adequate housing (Petersilia, 2003). Most ex-offenders are released to low-income, high-crime areas, where they live with family or friends who may not be supportive of abstinence. In many parts of the country the rates of reincarceration for parolees is extraordinarily high. For example, in California, two thirds of incarcerated offenders released on parole are reincarcerated within 3 years (Petersilia, 2003). Criminal justice research on parolees conducted by the Urban Institute (2006) suggests that the lack of satisfactory housing for offenders plays an important role in recidivism.

The enormous need for housing and recovery-related social support among individuals abstaining from alcohol and drug use makes a special edition of *JGAR* on Oxford House necessary and relevant. This introduction to that special edition sets a context for the articles that follow by reviewing studies that document the importance of social support and housing stability on recovery outcome. The focus then shifts to a review of the history of communal-living arrangements for alcoholics and addicts, starting with the early "dry hotels" or "lodging houses" (Wittman, 1993) and moving to contemporary abstinent living environments, such as sober living houses in California (Polcin, 2001; Polcin & Henderson, 2008) and sober houses on college campuses (Botzet, Winters, & Fahnhorst, in press; Laitman & Lederman, in press). Finally, the Oxford House model is briefly described in terms of its history, structure, and operations (see Jason, Ferrari, Davis, & Olson, 2006). After a review of recent research on outcomes in recovery-oriented communal-living environments, three conceptual views are presented as ways of understanding the improvements that residents make: (a) *social context theory* as described by Moos (2006), (b) *self-governance and self-care dynamics* as described by Khantzian and Mack (1994), and (c) *peer affiliation and identification* as described by Vaillant (1975). Several of the articles that follow in this special edition, in fact, expand on these concepts and more specifically depict their influence on the Oxford House model.

THE INFLUENCE OF SOCIAL SUPPORT AND HOUSING ON RECOVERY OUTCOME

A variety of studies have shown that social support relates to recovery. For example, Beattie and Longabaugh (1999) found that general social support, defined as having individuals in one's social network who provide a general sense of well-being, was associated with drinking outcome. However, alcohol-specific social support (i.e., encouragement to avoid drinking) appeared to be more strongly associated with outcome and longer periods of time (15 months, as opposed to 3 months for general social support).

Interventions for addiction that emphasize social support for recovery have received strong support in the outcome literature. For example, a number of studies conducted by Moos and colleagues (e.g., Moos & Moos, 2006) showed that involvement in Alcoholics Anonymous (AA) was strongly associated with positive outcome. Further, involvement in AA appeared to be associated with positive outcome for individuals involved in formal treatment as well as those in the general population.

A critically important part of an individual's social environment, however, is the person's living or housing situation. During the past 2 decades housing has become an increasingly important issue in the addiction outcome literature, in part because large proportions of individuals who are homeless have problems with drugs or alcohol (Robertson, Zlotnick, & Westerfelt, 1997; Wenzel, Ebener, Koegel, & Gelberg, 1996). In a number of studies, housing assistance and housing status were associated with treatment outcome (e.g., Bebout, Drake, Wie, McHugo, & Harris, 1997; Hitchcock et al., 1995; Milby et al., 1996; Miescher, & Galanter, 1996). Overall, these findings indicated that clients who were homeless or lived in substance-using environments during or after treatment were more prone to relapse than clients living in environments supportive of sobriety.

HISTORY OF COMMUNAL-LIVING ARRANGEMENTS
FOR INDIVIDUALS IN RECOVERY

Although the topic of housing received focus only recently in the addiction literature, individuals in recovery from addiction and professionals who work within this field have known that providing alcohol- and drug-free living environments is important. Some of the early efforts to create sober living environments were reviewed extensively elsewhere (i.e., Polcin, 2001; Polcin & Henderson, 2008) and are only briefly summarized in this article.

One of the earliest reviews of sober housing for alcoholics was provided by Wittman (1993). He noted that during the era of the Temperance Movement during the 1830s religious institutions, such as the YMCA and Salvation Army, developed "dry hotels" or "lodging houses" for alcoholics. These dwellings were designed to help individuals receive support for abstinence as well as exposure to religious instruction. The role of the residents in these facilities was quite different than that of Oxford House residents. Rather than being active participants in operations of the facilities (as in Oxford House, 2006; Ferrari, Jason, Olson, Davis, & Alvarez, 2002), they were generally quite passive. House rules and operations were developed by managers of the facilities, and residents were either required or strongly encouraged to attend religious services.

A second type of sober living facility developed during the late 1940s, after World War II, when Alcoholics Anonymous (AA) was becoming prominent and housing availability was limited (Wittman, 1993). In Los Angeles, recovering AA members opened "twelve step" houses to provide sober lodging to the growing number of alcoholics in the city. Managers of these houses either mandated or strongly encouraged attendance at AA meetings, and house operations were generally the responsibility or the house manager or owner. This passive role of house residents was similar to "dry hotels" or "lodging houses" and contrasts markedly with the active role of Oxford House residents (Ferrari, Jason, Davis, Olson, & Alvarez, 2004).

THE GROWING NEED FOR AFFORDABLE SOBER
LIVING ENVIRONMENTS

Despite the early efforts to provide sober living environments to alcoholics, the need for alcohol- and drug-free housing in the communities increased in recent years. The combination of cutbacks on publicly funded addiction treatment and tight housing markets resulted in an explosion of homelessness. As reviewed elsewhere (Polcin et al., 2004), homelessness affected nearly 6 million people from 1987 to 1993. Conservative estimates suggested about 40% of homeless suffered from alcohol problems and 15%

from drug problems (McCarty, Argeriou, Huebner, & Lubran, 1991). In one county in Northern California, for example, a study of homelessness revealed lifetime prevalence for substance use disorders of 69.1% (Robertson et al., 1997).

Two prominent factors fueled the need for affordable alcohol- and drug-free housing, namely, the deinstitutionalization of psychiatric hospitals over the last 4 decades (Polcin, 1990) and the explosion of the state and federal prison systems over the past 25 years (Petersilia, 2000, 2003). Neither individuals with psychiatric disorders leaving state psychiatric hospitals nor parolees transitioning from prison into the community received the services they needed (e.g., housing, employment, substance abuse, medical and mental health). Thus, few achieved stable lifestyles in the community and many became vulnerable to recidivism and homelessness (Fischer & Breakey, 1991; Petersilia, 2000, 2003).

CONTEMPORARY ABSTINENT LIVING ENVIRONMENTS

The need for drug- and alcohol-abstinent living environments overwhelms existing housing resources. However, a number of housing models are effective. In the addiction treatment field halfway or "step down" houses showed a great benefit for individuals leaving residential treatment programs as well as treatment programs for incarcerated offenders (Inciardi, 1996; Lockwood, Inciardi, & Surratt, 1997; Martin, Butzin, & Inciardi, 1995). Relative to individuals discharged into the community without supportive living environments, those men and women who found residence in halfway houses had better substance abuse, criminal justice and employment outcomes.

One problem with the halfway house model, however, is that lengths of stay are limited. A resident may have from several months to a year to adjust to life in the community and find alternative living arrangements. Frequently, pressures exist for residents to move out of a halfway house to open beds for others who seem to be more in need. Another criticism of the halfway house model is that they typically are financed using public funds and operated by professional staff within formal treatment systems. While some residents may require that level of structure and support, other individuals may benefit by taking on more responsibility and autonomy (Polcin, 2001; Polcin & Henderson, 2008).

California Sober Living Houses

California sober living houses (SLHs) avoid some of the problems that residents of halfway houses encounter. Unlike most halfway houses, they are financially self-sustaining such that government funding is not necessary.

Also, residents are free to remain at the facility for as long as they like, provided that they abide by house rules and pay rent. Although they originated in California during the 1970s, some SLH programs may be found in other states. As described in more detail elsewhere (Polcin, 2001), SLHs are based on a social model recovery philosophy that emphasizes abstinence and mutual help among residents.

Although there are similarities among California SLHs, there are important differences as well. For example, some SLHs implement social model recovery principles that emphasize empowering residents to be involved in house operations and management by participating in a democratically oriented residents' council. Other SLHs continue with a "strong manager" model of operations (Polcin & Henderson, 2008), similar to that used by the earlier "dry hotels" and "twelfth step" houses described above. A house manager or owner rents out rooms, collects money for rent and bills, evicts residents who relapse, and encourages or mandates attendance at 12-step meetings. Some of these houses are for-profit enterprises, prompting concern that they may be more focused on profit than recovery (Polcin, 2006a). Fortunately, several SLH coalitions emerged that either mandated or strongly encouraged houses to adopt social model principles into their programs, including mechanisms for resident input into house operations. These include the California Association of Addiction and Recovery Resources (CAARR) and the Sober Living Network (SLN). CAARR has about 64 member organizations that provide sober living services, and the SLN has over 260 sober living houses.

Although California model SLHs operated for decades, only recently have outcome evaluations been conducted. Polcin and Henderson (in press) reported outcomes of 130 individuals residing in 16 sober living houses in Northern California. Relative to their functioning before they entered the houses, residents made significant improvement on measures of alcohol and drug use, psychiatric symptoms, and employment. Forty percent of the individuals who entered the houses were completely abstinent over the 6-month assessment period, and an additional 24% were abstinent 5 of the 6 months. Among those persons who relapsed after entering the houses, there was a less severe pattern of substance use relative to their use before entering. As expected, one of the factors that correlated with improved outcome was higher involvement in 12-step recovery groups (Polcin & Henderson, 2008).

About a quarter of the residents in the SLHs were referred from the criminal justice system and had improvements similar to voluntary residents (Polcin, 2006b). The author pointed out that SLHs might be useful in playing a more prominent role in helping to reduce very serious overcrowding problems in state prisons, especially in California, where recidivism rates result in two thirds of state prison parolees being rearrested within 3 years.

College Dormitory Recovery Houses

A different model of sober housing was developed at Rutgers University in 1988 to address the needs of the growing number of college students with alcohol and drug problems (Botzet et al., in press; Laitman & Lederman, in press). Because of widespread drinking among students in the general population it was felt that separate dormitories designed for students in recovery would provide them emotional, social, and environmental support that would increase their chances at successful recovery. After recovery dormitories were implemented at Rutgers, 11 similar recovery dormitories have been developed at on other college campuses. Unlike California SLHs, students can only reside in the dormitories while they are students at the college. Although peer support for recovery is emphasized, these living arrangements are integrated into an overall treatment approach that requires regular sessions with alcohol and drug counselors on campus (Laitman & Lederman, in press).

THE OXFORD HOUSE MODEL

The largest organized model of providing alcohol- and drug-free housing in communal-living environments is *Oxford House*. Currently, there are over 1,200 houses throughout the United States, Canada, and Australia. All houses are gender specific and located in quiet, middle-class neighborhoods (Ferrari, Jason, Sasser, Davis, & Olson, 2006). Although Oxford Houses do not require any specific involvement in treatment or 12-step groups, many residents are involved in these types of services. For example, Nealon-Woods, Ferrari, and Jason (1995) found that 76% of a sample of 134 male residents in Oxford Houses attended 12-step meetings at least weekly. Like the 12-step model of recovery, Oxford Houses adopt a goal of abstinence, and substance use while residing in an Oxford House is grounds for discharge (Ferrari et al., 2004). As the subsequent articles in this special edition show, Oxford Houses have been effective with a range of populations.

The origins of Oxford House set the direction for the housing model that followed. Briefly, after a halfway house operated by a treatment provider in Silver Spring, Maryland, closed, the residents continued living there by paying rent and bills themselves. They agreed to support each other in the recovery process and mandated that any use of substances by a resident would require that they leave. They did not mandate any involvement in treatment or attendance at AA; those decisions were left to the residents themselves (Davis, Olson, Jason, Alvarez, & Ferrari, 2006). Residents were apparently satisfied with this arrangement and houses began expanding. The pace of expansion increased when a federal law was passed (Public Law 100-690) which required states to loan money to individuals or groups for start-up costs associated with alcohol- and drug-free residences. For a more detailed description of the history of Oxford Houses see O'Neill (1990) or Jason et al. (2006).

The Oxford House model of communal recovery housing offers a number of advantages over traditional modes of treatment. Oxford Houses are readily replicable (Ferrari et al., 2004, 2006). The *Oxford House Manual* (2006) describes specific requirements for how many individuals may live in a house, minimum amount of square footage, and types of neighborhood where they can be established. Because all costs are covered by residents, Oxford Houses may be immune to many external threats that detrimentally affect treatment programs (e.g., managed care models of funding).

A particular advantage of the Oxford House model is that guidelines provided by the *Oxford House Manual* (2006) stipulated the use of organizational principles consistent with a social model philosophy of recovery. For example, all houses are rental properties, and management of house operations requires a shared, rotating leadership structure (Ferrari, Jason, Blake, Davis, & Olson, 2006). Thus, a "strong manager" type of house with one person in a position of authority is not possible (Jason, Braciszewski, Olson, & Ferrari, 2005). Each member of the house takes responsibility for paying rent and meeting household costs (Ferrari et al., 2004). This opportunity for shared responsibility and empowerment within a communal-living environment is an integral part of the philosophy of recovery (Ferrari et al., 2002).

Outcome Research

Leonard Jason, Joe Ferrari, and their research group at DePaul University conducted a wide range of studies on Oxford Houses over the past 14 years that culminated in a recent book *Creating Communities for Addiction Recovery* (Jason et al., 2006). Many of their Oxford House studies were reviewed in the articles that follow. Here, I examine two major analyses of long-term outcomes of Oxford House residents.

The first study, Jason, Olson, Ferrari, and Lo Sasso (2006), examined 150 individuals completing residential treatment programs. Half these participants were randomly assigned to usual aftercare and half to Oxford Houses. At 24-month follow up, individuals assigned to the Oxford House condition had significantly better outcome on measures of substance use, income, and incarceration. One limitation of that study, however, was that all Oxford Houses were located in Illinois. A second limitation was their study findings might only be generalized to individuals completing residential treatment.

The second outcome study, Jason, Davis, Ferrari, and Anderson (2007), circumvented both of these concerns. A large, national U.S. sample of Oxford House residents was recruited ($N = 897$) without respect to treatment history. Oxford House residents were recruited into the study and interviewed at three 4-month intervals. Rates of abstinence during the final interview were high. About 13.5% of the respondents reported using alcohol or drugs in the past 90 days. Consistent with social model recovery philosophy, social support for sobriety was associated with abstinence. A second important finding was the high rate at which residents found employment. Throughout the course of the study employment ranged from 79% to 86%.

Conceptual Perspectives on How Oxford Houses Help

The growth and success of Oxford Houses begs the question of how they help residents. This section will attempt to conceptualize how Oxford Houses help by briefly identifying three conceptual perspectives: social context, self-governance and self-care, and peer affiliation and identification.

A number of articles that follow in this special edition expand upon these three general frameworks. For example, social context and peer factors in Oxford Houses are addressed by Graham, Jason, and Ferrari (this issue) in their report on "psychological sense of community." An article by Viola, Ferrari, Davis, and Jason (this issue) examines peer influences in terms of the role and prevalence of helping others among Oxford House residents. Groh, Jason, and Ferrari (this issue) present data depicting how 12-step involvement interacts with the social environment within Oxford Houses to produce better outcomes. Intrapsychic issues relevant to Oxford House residents are addressed as well. For example, Ferrari et al. (this issue) describe a study on self-regulation among Oxford House residents and report that it is associated with length of sobriety. A number of articles in this edition describe recovery for specific populations of Oxford House residents, such as women with children, criminal justice–involved individuals, and ethnic minorities. Future articles might examine how the dynamics of change for these groups are similar and different to the larger population of Oxford House residents.

SOCIAL CONTEXT

A recent article by Moos (2006) summarized the social context perspective on substance use and recovery by emphasizing four related theories: social control, behavioral economics, social learning, and stress and coping. Each has implications for understanding what is helpful to residents of Oxford Houses.

Social control refers to the bonds that individuals have with family, school, work, and other social institutions that can help shield them from substance use. These relationships motivate individuals to engage in prosocial behaviors that contribute to the community and refrain from antisocial and destructive behaviors. Social organization, structure, cohesion, and monitoring behavior all contribute to social control. Within Oxford Houses, the social bonds that residents have with each other, the larger recovery community, and mutual-help groups such as Alcoholics Anonymous help shield them from relapse. Although Oxford Houses allow for substantial autonomy among residents, there are some clear structures and guidelines that facilitate recovery-oriented behaviors, social organization, and cohesion. Examples of social control within Oxford Houses include monitoring residents' sobriety, requiring that residents take part in house meetings and leadership positions, and implementing house and regional social events that build cohesion among residents.

The second social context theory is *behavioral economics*, which is closely related to social control theory. It addressed the question of what behaviors are reinforcing for individuals. Is the individual engaged in non-substance activities that they experience as reinforcing? For individuals attempting recovery from addiction, have they learned to meet their physical, emotional, and social needs in ways that do not involve substance use or related behaviors? Residence in an Oxford House exposes residents to alternative ways of getting their needs met that substitute for alcohol and drug use. Some aspects of the environment are reinforcing in and of themselves, such as general social support, support for sobriety, and recreational activities that are shared among residents. For many residents, the requirement that they be involved in decision making and leadership positions in the house is reinforcing in terms of building self-esteem and a sense of self-efficacy. Residents also provide each other with suggestions and resources for alternative ways of getting needs met.

The third aspect of Moos's (2006) social context perspective on addiction is *social learning* theory. He suggests that adult and peer role models play strong roles in the development of addiction problems that typically begin in adolescence. Similarly, role models play important roles in recovery. Oxford Houses provide a peer-focused model of recovery, where new residents learn from those with more recovery experience. In addition to adapting recovery behaviors modeled, residents also adopt attitudes and norms that support a recovery lifestyle.

Stress and coping theory is the final component to Moos's view of how the social context influences the onset of addiction as well as recovery from it. Essentially, individuals use substances in response to stressful life circumstances, some of which are exacerbated by social disorganization within institutions and neighborhoods. One advantage of residence in Oxford Houses is that in general they tend to be located in middle-class areas that are not high in crime or drug use. This helps decrease stress and the potential for relapse. Beyond that, residents role model stress management strategies for each other, and they share recovery resources for managing stress.

A different way of conceptualizing how Oxford Houses help comes from the work of Khantzian and Mack (1994), who emphasized how self-governance and self-care can be enhanced within a supportive group of recovering individuals. Although their article addressed how addicts and alcoholics change in Alcoholics Anonymous meetings, many of the concepts presented also apply to other group environments, such as Oxford Houses.

Rather than emphasizing processes within the social environment that lead directly to behavioral change, Khantzian and Mack (1994) explored how the social environment affects internal emotional states that frequently lead to substance use. They noted that many individuals suffering from addiction have powerful emotional experiences that they have difficulty managing and that leave them vulnerable to relapse. The authors suggested the external support provided by AA helped compensate for internal vulnerability. In addition, the honest sharing of life stories in AA facilitated self-examination and self-expression among individuals who otherwise would not examine their internal states, let alone share them with others. The support and understanding that frequently takes place as members tell their stories provides powerful corrective experiences. In addition, sharing stories also helps other members heal some of their affective deficits through identification with the speaker. Over time, AA members are able to develop more mature and flexible management of the affective states.

Residence in an Oxford House is separate from being a member of AA. However, many of the mechanisms through which people are helped may be similar. Albeit more informally than in an AA meeting, Oxford House residents nonetheless often share their addiction and recovery stories with each other in ways that might be similarly helpful. In addition, the social support and structure within the houses may help residents manage their emotional states more effectively, particularly in terms of not using substances to manage them. Finally, as with the AA fellowship, there is frequently an experience of being part of something larger than oneself that is reassuring and helps contain powerful affect.

The role of human relationships in helping AA members govern their feelings and care for themselves without resorting to substance use seems equally applicable to the Oxford House setting: "AA stresses the importance of human interdependence. It replaces a chemical solution for disordered impulses, distress, and suffering with a human one," (Khantzian & Mack, 1994, p. 90).

SELF-GOVERNANCE AND SELF-CARE

Peer Affiliation or Identification

Over 30 years ago Vaillant (1975) described how peer relationships were vital to successful transition out of drug addiction. Although his article technically addressed sociopathy, Vaillant (1975) noted that many narcotic addicts often presented similar symptoms and responded to similar interventions. He suggested that external control over drug use and related behaviors that were destructive to self and others was a prerequisite of recovery. Many individuals with sociopathy or addiction problems were thought to be incapable of modifying destructive and antisocial behaviors on their own. Thus, therapists who did not provide containing interventions left these clients feeling abandoned. Vaillant (1975) suggested residential treatment settings could provide the containment needed by implementing "realistic but not punitive" (p. 178) confrontation of the consequences of their behavior.

For Valliant, antisocial behaviors were viewed in part as attempts avoid anxiety and flee from human intimacy, which was experienced as frightening. Only when such behaviors were thwarted could the client be open to the type of honest human encounter that facilitates recovery. Finally, Valliant suggested that conventional individual therapy was not sufficient for individuals with narcotic addiction. The paths out of addiction were believed to be like the paths out of adolescence; they came from identification with peers (Valliant, 1975).

While Oxford houses do not offer the intensive level of supervision that Valliant advocated, they do offer containment over destruction behaviors by providing peer-administered consequences in response to them. In addition, Oxford Houses provide peer pressures to avoid destructive behaviors such as substance use. Any use of substances while residing in an Oxford house is explicitly prohibited and is grounds for eviction. Other destructive behaviors are prohibited as well, such as acts of violence and theft. Resident-imposed penalties for proscribed behaviors and can range from eviction, to a written contract mandating improvement, to a fine.

Although sanctions for destructive behaviors are important, the sense of belonging to something larger may be an equally potent way that Oxford Houses contain destructive behaviors. Oxford Houses offer an invitation to their residents to take part in a community of recovering individuals that provides a sense of social support, understanding, empowerment, and nurturing that has been absent from the lives of many. The identification and affiliation that Oxford House residents develop with peers who similarly struggle with inclinations to run from their anxiety, affect, and feelings of intimacy provides the groundwork for the path out of addiction and into recovery.

CONCLUSION

Although a variety of treatment and self-help approaches for addiction have been shown to be effective, many individuals are unable to sustain the improvements they make because they are unable to find living environments that support their recovery. Housing costs in the United States and elsewhere have made matters worse by driving addicts and alcoholics with limited resources into high-crime areas where they are likely to relapse. Vulnerable populations, such as criminal justice offenders and individuals with psychiatric disorders, have a particularly difficult time finding alcohol- and drug-free housing, and they comprise large proportions of the homeless.

All of these conditions make this special edition on Oxford Houses timely and significant. Although a variety different communal housing models have been used to provide alcohol- and drug-free housing to individuals suffering from addiction, none are currently more popular or widespread than the Oxford House model. Oxford Houses have the advantages of being financially independent, peer managed, and easily replicable. Outcome studies have shown they can be effective for a variety of individuals.

Research on Oxford Houses to date has documented positive longitudinal outcomes. Confirming an important part of the recovery philosophy, studies have also found that social support for sobriety is associated with better outcome. However, more research is needed on the mechanisms of how Oxford Houses affect positive change in residents. It would be particularly interesting to examine variations in the social environments of houses and correlate social environment characteristics with outcomes.

Three different ways of conceptualizing how residents improve have been presented: social context, self-governance and self-care, and peer affiliation and identification. The ways in which a number of the articles that follow in this special edition expand on these perspectives have been described, and a suggestion has been made to address whether specific populations within Oxford Houses have similar or different mechanisms of change compared to the overall population of residents.

REFERENCES

Beattie, M., & Longabaugh, R. (1999). General and alcohol-specific social support following treatment. *Addictive Behaviors, 24,* 593–606.

Bebout, R. R., Drake, R. E., Wie, H., McHugo, G. J., & Harris, M. (1997). Housing status among formerly homeless dually diagnosed adults. *Psychiatric Services, 48,* 963–941.

Botzet, A., Winters, K., & Fahnhorst, T. (in press). An exploratory assessment of a college substance abuse recovery program: Augsburg College's StepUP program. *Journal on Groups in Addiction and Recovery.*

Davis, M. I., Olson, B., Jason, L. A., Alvarez, J., & Ferrari, J. R. (2006). Cultivating and maintaining effective action research partnerships: The DePaul and Oxford House collaborative. *Journal of Prevention & Intervention in the Community, 31,* 3–12.

Ferrari, J. R., Jason, L. A., Davis, M. I., Olson, B. D., & Alvarez, J. (2004). Similarities and differences in governance among residents in drug and/or alcohol misuse:

Self vs. staff rules and regulations. *Therapeutic Communities: The International Journal for Therapeutic and Supportive Organizations, 25*, 179–192.

Ferrari, J. R., Jason, L. A., Olson, B. D., Davis, M., & Alvarez, J. (2002). Sense of community among Oxford House residents recovering from substance abuse: Making a house a home. In A. T. Fischer, C. C. Sonn, & B. J. Bishop (Eds.), *Psychological sense of community: Research, applications, and implications* (pp. 109–122). New York: Kluwer/Plenum.

Ferrari, J. R., Jason, L. A., Blake, R., Davis, M. I., & Olson, B. D. (2006). "This is my neighborhood": Comparing United States and Australian Oxford House neighborhoods. *Journal of Prevention & Intervention in the Community, 31*, 41–50.

Ferrari, J. R., Jason, L. A., Sasser, K. C., Davis, M. I., & Olson, B. D. (2006). Creating a home to promote recovery: The physical environments of Oxford House. *Journal of Prevention & Intervention in the Community, 31*, 27–40.

Fischer, P. J., & Breakey, W. R. (1991). The epidemiology of alcohol, drugs, and mental disorders among homeless persons. *American Psychologist, 46*, 1115–1128.

Graham, B., Jason, L., & Ferrari, J. (this issue). Sense of community within recovery housing: Impact of resident age and income. *Journal of Groups in Addiction and Recovery*.

Groh, B., Jason, L., & Ferrari, J. (this issue). Oxford House and Alcoholics Anonymous: The impact of mutual help models on abstinence. *Journal of Groups in Addiction and Recovery*.

Hitchcock, H. C., Stainback, R. D., & Roque, G. M. (1995). Effects of halfway house placement on retention of patients in substance abuse aftercare. *American Journal of Drug and Alcohol Abuse, 21*, 379–390.

Inciardi, J. A. (1996). Therapeutic Community: An effective model for corrections-based drug abuse treatment. In K. E. Early (Ed.), *Drug treatment behind bars: Prison-based strategies for change* (pp. 65–74). Westport, CT: Praeger.

Jason, L. A., Braciszewski, J., Olson, B. D., & Ferrari, J. R. (2005). Increasing the number of mutual help recovery homes for substance abusers: Effects of government policy and funding assistance. *Behavioral and Social Issues, 14*, 71–79.

Jason, L. A., Davis, M. I., Ferrari, J. R., & Anderson, E. (2007). The need for substance abuse after-care: A longitudinal analysis of Oxford House. *Addictive Behaviors, 32*, 803–818.

Jason, L., Ferrari, J., Davis, M., & Olson, B. (2006). *Creating communities for addiction recovery*. New York: Haworth Press.

Jason, L. A., Olson, B. D., Ferrari, J. R., & Lo Sasso, A. T. (2006). Communal housing settings enhance substance abuse recovery. *American Journal of Public Health, 91*, 1727–1729.

Khantzian, E. J., & Mack J. E. (1994). How AA works and why it's important for clinicians to understand. *Journal of Substance Abuse Treatment, 11*(2), 77–92.

Laitman, L., & Lederman, L. (in press). The need for a continuum of care: The Rutgers comprehensive model. *Journal on Groups in Addiction and Recovery*.

Lockwood, D., Inciardi, J. A., & Surratt, H. L. (1997). CREST Outreach Center: A model for blending treatment and corrections. In F. M. Tims, J. A. Inciardi, B. W. Fletcher, and A. M. Horton Jr. (Eds.), *Effectiveness of innovative approaches in the treatment of drug abuse* (pp. 70–82). Westport, CT: Greenwood.

Martin, S. S., Butzin, C. A., & Inciardi, J. A. (1995). Assessment of a multistage therapeutic community for drug-involved offenders. *Journal of Psychoactive Drugs, 27*(1), 106–116.

McCarty, D., Argeriou, M., Huebner, R. B., & Lubran, B. (1991). Alcoholism, drug abuse, and the homeless [Special issue: Homelessness]. *American Psychologist, 46*(11), 1139–1148.

Milby, J. B., Schumacher, J. E., Wallace, D., Feedman, M. J., & Vuchinich, R. E. (1996). To house or not to house: The effects of providing housing to home-less substance abusers in treatment. *American Journal of Public Health, 95*(7), 1259–1265.

Miescher, A., & Galanter, M. (1996). Shelter-based treatment of the homeless alco-holic. *Journal of Substance Abuse Treatment, 13*(2), 135–140.

Moos, R. H. (2006). Social contexts and substance use. In W. R. Miller and K. M. Carroll. (Eds.), *Substance abuse: What the science tells us and what we should do about it* (pp. 182–200). New York: Guilford.

Moos, R. H., & Moos, B. S. (2006). Treated and untreated individuals with alcohol use disorders: Rates and predictors of remission and relapse. *International Journal of Clinical and Health Psychology, 6*(3), 513–526.

National Institute on Drug Abuse (NIDA). (1999). *Principles of drug addiction treat-ment: A research based guide* (NIH Publication No. 00-4180). Bethesda, MD: Author.

Nealon-Woods, M. A., Ferrari, J. R., & Jason, L. A. (1995). Twelve-step program use among Oxford House residents: Spirituality or social support in sobriety? *Journal of Substance Abuse, 7*(3), 311–318.

O'Neill, J. (1990). History of Oxford House, Inc. In S. Shaw & T. Borkman. (Eds.), *Social model recovery: An environmental approach* (pp. 103–107). Burbank, CA: Bridge Focus.

Oxford House. (2006 September). *Oxford House manual.* Silver Spring, MD: Author.

Petersilia, J. (2000). When prisoners return to the community: Political, economic, and social consequence. *Sentencing and Corrections, 9*, 1–8.

Petersilia, J. (2003). *When prisoners come home: Parole and prisoner reentry.* New York: Oxford University Press.

Polcin, D. L. (1990). Administrative planning in community mental health. *Commu-nity Mental Health Journal, 26*(2), 181–192.

Polcin, D. L. (2001). Sober living houses: Potential roles in substance abuse services and suggestions for research. *Substance Use and Misuse, 36*(2), 301–311.

Polcin, D. L. (2006a). How health services research can help clinical trials become more community relevant. *International Journal of Drug Policy, 17*(3), 230–237.

Polcin, D. L. (2006b). What about Sober Living Houses for parolees? *Criminal Justice Studies: A Critical Journal of Crime Law and society, 19*(3), 291–300.

Polcin, D. L., & Henderson, D. (2008). A clean and sober place to live: Philosophy, structure, and purported therapeutic factors in sober living houses. *Journal of Psychoactive Drugs, 40*(2), 153–159.

Polcin, D. L., Galloway, G. P., Taylor, K., & Benowitz-Fredericks (2004). Why we need to study sober living houses. *Counselor: The Magazine for Addiction Professionals, 5*(5), 36–45.

Robertson, M. J., Zlotnick, C., & Westerfelt, A. (1997). Drug use disorders and treatment contact among homeless adults in Alameda County, California. *American Journal of Public Health, 87*(2), 221–228.

Urban Institute. (2006, January). *Understanding the challenges of prisoner reentry: Research findings from the Urban Institute's Prisoner Reentry Portfolio.* Washington, DC: Justice Policy Center.

Vaillant, G. E. (1975). Sociopathy as a human process: A viewpoint. *Archives of General Psychiatry, 32*(2), 178–183.

Viola, J., Ferrari, J., Davis, M., & Jason, L. (this issue). Measuring in-group and out-group helping in communal living: Helping and substance abuse recovery. *Journal of Groups in Addiction and Recovery.*

Wenzel, S. L., Ebener, P. A., Koegel, P., & Gelberg, L. (1996). Drug-abusing homeless clients in California's substance abuse treatment system. *Journal of Psychoactive Drugs, 28*(2), 147–159.

Wittman, F. D. (1993). Affordable housing for people with alcohol and other drug problems. *Contemporary Drug Problems, 20*(3), 541–609.

Oxford House and Alcoholics Anonymous: The Impact of Two Mutual-Help Models on Abstinence

DAVID R. GROH, PhD, LEONARD A. JASON, PhD, and
JOSEPH R. FERRARI, PD

DePaul University

MARGARET I. DAVIS, PhD

Dickinson College

Two examples of mutual-help approaches for substance abuse recovery are 12-step groups (AA and NA) and Oxford House. The present study examined the combined effects of AA and Oxford House residence on abstinence over a 24-month period, with 150 individuals randomly assigned to either an Oxford House or to usual aftercare. Among individuals with high 12-step involvement, the addition of Oxford House residence significantly increased the odds of abstinence (87.5% vs. 52.9%). However, among participants with low 12-step involvement, rates of abstinence were fairly similar across conditions (31.4% vs. 21.2%). Results suggested that the joint effectiveness of these mutual-help programs may promote abstinence.

From a public policy perspective, understanding how mutual-help groups and self-help treatments might be alternatives to professional aftercare programs seems important (Humphreys, 2004; Tonigan, Toscova, & Miller, 1996). Unlike traditional treatments programs, self-help or mutual-help groups represent voluntarily gathered social support assemblies working together on a common problem with self-directed leadership and the sharing

The authors appreciate the financial support from the National Institute on Alcohol Abuse and Alcoholism (grant number AA12218).

of experiences (Humphreys, 2004). In general, self-help therapy was more effective and less expensive than traditional, professional-focused therapy (Humphreys, 2004). The best-known example of mutual-help groups supporting abstinence is the *12-step program*, which includes groups such as *Alcoholics Anonymous (AA)* and *Narcotics Anonymous* (*NA*; McCrady & Miller, 1993).

Alcoholics Anonymous was created in 1935 as a self-help group for individuals in alcohol recovery to maintain sobriety through spirituality, social support, and progression through 12-step treatment. Today, more people turn to AA to recover from alcohol addiction than any other program (McCrady & Miller, 1993; Weisner, Greenfield, & Room, 1995), with worldwide membership estimated at over 2 million in 150 countries (Alcoholics Anonymous, 2006). Members progress toward recovery at their own pace through the sharing of experience, hope, and strength, admitting powerlessness over alcohol through self-disclosure at each of 12 steps (Emrick, Tonigan, Montgomery, & Little, 1993). Unlike conventional alcohol treatments, AA is not time limited, lacks professional involvement, charges no dues or fees, and keeps no membership lists at weekly meetings (Kurtz, 1979).

Numerous studies found AA participation related to improved alcohol use outcomes (e.g., Longabaugh, Wirtz, Zweben, & Stout, 1998; Montgomery, Miller, & Tonigan, 1995; Ouimette, Moos, & Finney, 1998; Pisani, Fawcett, Clark, & McGuire, 1993). Meta-analyses of AA effectiveness studies concluded that participation related to positive drinking outcomes and better psychological health, social functioning, employment situation, and legal situation (Emrick et al., 1993; Tonigan et al., 1996). Still, there is a general lack of longitudinal research exploring effectiveness of these programs (Humphreys, 2004), and researchers continue to debate the rigor and quality of AA outcome studies (Emrick et al., 1993; Humphreys, 2004; McCrady & Miller, 1993; Kownacki & Shadish, 1999).

Another mutual help–founded intervention for substance abuse based on a network of community-based recovery homes is called *Oxford House* (*OH*). OH was established in 1975 for persons who seek a supportive, mutual-help, residential setting with recovering peers in order to develop long-term sobriety skills (Jason, Davis, Ferrari, & Bishop, 2001). To date, there are over 1,250 dwellings across the USA, Canada, and Australia. Similar to AA, OH may be more cost effective than other aftercare treatments because each House group is financially self-supported, and no professionals are involved. Each house is a rented, multibedroom dwelling for same-sex occupants, located in low-crime residential neighborhoods (see Ferrari et al., this issue). Houses operate democratically by majority rule, governed by house officers who are elected every 6 months (Oxford House, 2002). Residents may stay in an OH indefinitely, given that they avoid substance use and disruptive behavior.

Regarding the effectiveness of Oxford House, results of follow-up assessments of residents from 6 to 24 months found that 62–69% of residents either remained in the house or left on good terms (Bishop, Jason, Ferrari, & Huang, 1998; Majer, Jason, Ferrari, & North, 2002). In addition, a large nationwide 12-month longitudinal study found that length of stay in Oxford predicted social support, self-efficacy, and abstinence (Jason, Davis, Ferrari, & Anderson, 2007). Jason, Olson, Ferrari, & Lo Sasso (2006) reported a randomized study that compared Oxford House residents with participants in usual aftercare settings. At a 2-year follow up, Oxford House residents had lower substance use (31% vs. 65%, respectively), higher monthly income ($989 vs. $440), and lower incarceration rates (3% vs. 9%).

The Oxford House organization encourages 12-step participation (Oxford House, 2002), and most residents are involved in AA or NA (Flynn, Alvarez, Jason, Olson, Ferrari, & Davis, 2006; Nealon-Woods, Ferrari, & Jason, 1995). In addition, Majer, Jason, Ferrari, Venable, and Olson (2002) reported that time spent in Oxford House, combined with 12-step participation, related to increased levels of abstinence social support and abstinence self-efficacy. However, none of these studies jointly examined AA and OH models with the same individuals. Both mutual-help programs may individually promote recovery through emphasis on positive social support, strict rules, abstinent living, and self-direction; alternatively, a combination of OH and 12-step groups might produce the most positive outcomes. The present study assessed how involvement in Oxford House *and* 12-step groups related to abstinence among individuals in substance abuse recovery randomly assigned into Oxford House or usual care conditions.

METHOD

Procedure

We examined data from a longitudinal assessment of 150 individuals in substance abuse recovery from Northern Illinois (see Jason et al., 2006). In the present study, individuals discharged from residential substance abuse treatment facilities were randomly assigned to either a democratic, self-run, recovery home condition (Oxford House; $n = 75$) or to a usual aftercare condition ($n = 75$). The control comparison condition of usual care provided clients with several options prior to discharge, including referral to different forms of outpatient treatment, referral to self-help groups, or referral to other resources in the community.

All participants completed a baseline questionnaire assessment 2 to 3 days before discharge from inpatient substance abuse treatment programs. After participants entered the study, they were assessed every 6 months over a 2-year period, creating a total of five assessments (i.e., baseline, 6, 12, 18, and 24 months), and paid $40 at each interview wave.

Measures

We obtained baseline demographic information (e.g., gender, race, substance disorder typology) from items on the fifth edition of the Addiction Severity Index—Lite (ASI; McLellan et al., 1992). The ASI assessed common problems related to substance abuse: medical status, drug use, alcohol use, illegal activity, family relations, and psychiatric condition. This inventory was used in a number of alcohol and drug use studies over the past 15 years with excellent predictive and concurrent validities (McLellan et al., 1993).

The *Form 90* (Miller & Del Boca, 1994) obtained a continuous record of alcohol and drug consumption and intensity within a 90-day time span. This measure gathered information related to employment, health care utilization, incarceration, and alcohol and other drug use over a 90-day retrospective (a reliable time frame for abstinence assessment; Miller & Del Boca, 1994). Test–retest reliability was excellent for core variables, including total consumption (0.91–0.97), drinks per day (0.88–0.93), percent days abstinent (0.96–0.98), and percent heavy drinking days (0.92–0.97). Even though this study employed 6-month assessment intervals, Form 90 captured substance usage and 12-step participation during the last 90 days of each 6-month period.

RESULTS

Baseline Sociodemographic Analyses

No significant differences were found between the Oxford House and usual care conditions on baseline sociodemographic variables (Jason et al., 2006). Across both conditions, most participants were women (62%). As for ethnic status, this sample consisted of 77.3% African American, 11.3% Caucasian, 8% Hispanic/Latino, and 3.3% others. The average participant was 37.1 ($SD = 8.1$) years old and had 12.0 ($SD = 2.1$) years of education. With regards to marital status, 60.5% were never married; 26.5% were divorced, widowed, or separated; and 12.9% were married. Regarding psychological status, 59.3% had a lifetime Axis I Mood or Anxiety disorder, and 27.6% reported a lifetime history of having been prescribed psychological medications. In terms of legal history, 43.9% of participants had been incarcerated at some point, with an average of 2.9 ($SD = 7.3$) lifetime incarcerations. In the 6 months prior to the start of the study, 93.3% of participants had used alcohol or drugs.

Chi-square Analyses for Condition and 12-step Involvement

One participant was dropped from the following analyses due to reporting extreme and almost certainly false data regarding 12-step involvement along

TABLE 1 Chi-Squares for 12-Step Involvement by Condition across Different Time Intervals

| Time interval | % participating in 12-step groups | | |
	Oxford House condition	Usual Care condition	*Pearson chi-square*
0-6 months	91	79	3.81*
6-12 months	83	82	.02
12-18 months	88	63	10.57**
18-24 months	78	65	2.75
Entire course of study	95	89	1.45

$n = 149.$; *$p \leq .05$; **$p \leq .01$.

with other treatment variables. Table 1 shows the percentages in each condition participating in 12-step programs at each wave of data collection. At each time period, more individuals in the Oxford House condition attended 12-step groups than usual care. Chi-square analyses (condition [Oxford House or usual care] by 12-step participation [any or none]) indicated that this difference in utilization between Oxford House and usual care participants was significant during the 0–6 and 12–18 month periods of the study.

For all subsequent analyses, we dichotomized 12-step participation with a median split for several reasons. Since the Form 90 only assesses 12-step participation over a 90-day period, whereas data collections took place at 6-month intervals, we did not have a complete and continuous record of meetings attended over the course of the study. Also, because almost all participants attended at least a few 12-step meetings throughout the study, it would not be very meaningful to compare individuals who attended 12-step meetings with those who attended no meetings; thus, a median split divided 12-step involvement into high versus low (i.e., greater or less than 154 meetings attended during the study). This practice is supported in substance abuse literature, as previous studies have used related classifications of AA involvement (e.g., Alford, Koehler, & Leonard, 1991; Snow, Prochaska, & Rossi, 1994; Wallace, McNeill, Gilfillan, MacLean, & Fanella, 1988).

TABLE 2 Chi-Squares for 24-month Abstinence by 12-step Involvement during Study

| Condition | Low 12-step involvement | | High 12-step involvement | | Pearson chi-square |
	% abstinent	n	% abstinent	n	
Oxford House	31.4	35	87.5	40	10.3*
Usual Care	21.2	40	52.9	34	24.7*
Pearson chi-square	2.0		10.8*		

$n = 149$; *$p \leq .001$.

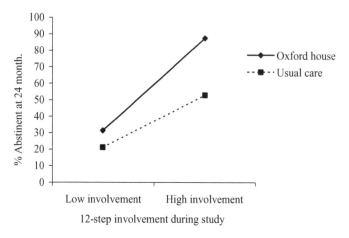

FIGURE 1 Interaction between condition and 12-step involvement during the study as related to rates of abstinence at the 24-month assessment.

Table 2 reports 24-month abstinence rates based on condition (Oxford House vs. usual care) and 12-step participation (high vs. low) during the course of the study. Overall, Oxford House participants had higher 24-month abstinence rates than usual care participants, and the high 12-step participation group had higher rates compared to the low participation group. Chi-square analyses (abstinence [yes or no] by 12-step participation [high or low]) indicated that for both Oxford House (X^2 [1, $N = 75$] $= 24.75, p = .000$) and usual care conditions (X^2 [1, $N = 74$] $= 10.32, p = .001$), abstinence rates were significantly higher among those with high 12-step participation. In addition, chi-square analyses (abstinence [yes or no] by condition [Oxford House or usual care]) demonstrated that among individuals with high 12-step involvement (X^2 [1, $N = 74$] $= 10.80, p = .001$), abstinence rates were significantly higher among Oxford House compared to usual care participants. However, no significant difference concerning abstinence was found between conditions among participants who were less involved in 12-step groups. Figure 1 illustrates this interaction effect.

DISCUSSION

Public health officials interested in mutual-help groups and self-help treatments explored alternative programs to professional treatment aftercare (Humphreys, 2004; Tonigan et al., 1996). In this study we provided the first systematic examination of two such mutual-help models for substance abuse treatment: 12-groups (i.e., AA) and a communal-living recovery model (OH). Given OH's emphasis on 12-step involvement (Oxford House, 2002), it was not surprising that OH residents attended more 12-step meetings than did usual care participants. At each time period, the majority of OH residents (between 78 and 95%) participated in these recovery groups. usual care participant rates in 12-step programs were similar but slightly lower (79 to 89%). Thus, one benefit of OH may be promoting 12-step utilization.

Looking at these two mutual-help programs separately, participants with high 12-step participation consistently had higher 24-month abstinence rates than participants with low participation. In fact, regardless of condition, participants who attended more 12-step meetings reported more than twice the likelihood of being abstinent than individuals who attended fewer meetings. This result was consistent with previous research on AA participation and improved alcohol use outcomes (e.g., Emrick et al., 1993; Longabaugh et al., 1998; Montgomery et al., 1995; Ouimette et al., 1998; Pisani et al., 1993; Tonigan et al., 1996). Oxford House residents also had higher abstinence rates overall than usual aftercare participants, consistent with past research (see Jason et al., 2006).

Regarding the combined impact of these programs, OH residents who were more involved in AA and NA had the highest rates of abstinence at 24 months (87.5%). Furthermore, the lowest rates of abstinence were reported among usual care participants with low 12-step involvement (21.2%). While abstinence rates did not differ significantly between conditions, among high 12-step attendees, OH residents had a major advantage over usual care participants. A combination of these two mutual-help programs might have produced the best outcomes for OH residents because of the joint emphasis on positive social support, strict rules, abstinent living, and self-direction. These two programs offered adults in recovery settings to develop a strong sense of community with similar others who share common abstinence goals (Ferrari et al., 2002). Receiving support for abstinence, guidance, and information from others committed to maintaining long-term recovery may enable addicts to avoid relapse.

There were several limitations of this study. Those participants assigned to the OH condition were brought to the Houses by the recruiters to ensure that they were actually included in that condition, whereas the usual care participants did not have this additional support. Future studies might provide equal support to adults in usual aftercare conditions to ensure equivalent contact with research staff. Also, while collateral report data confirmed self-reports of abstinence, biological confirmations of abstinence were not utilized in the present study. We also chose to dichotomize our variables in order to study the effects of either utilizing or not utilizing these mutual-help recovery tools (i.e., OH and 12-step programs); future studies may utilize continuous data to answer these questions to produce greater variability and ability to detect effects. Nonetheless, results of this study clearly point toward the joint effectiveness of these two mutual-help programs in promoting abstinence.

REFERENCES

Alford, G. S., Koehler, R. A., & Leonard, J. (1991). Alcoholics Anonymous–Narcotics Anonymous model inpatient treatment of chemically dependent adolescents: A 2-year outcome study. *Journal of Studies on Alcohol, 52,* 118–126.

Bishop, P. D., Jason, L. A., Ferrari, J. R., & Huang, C. F. (1998). A survival analysis of communal living, self-help, addiction recovery participants. *American Journal of Community Psychology, 26,* 803–821.

Emrick, C. D., Tonigan, J. S., Montgomery, H., & Little, L. (1993). Alcoholics anonymous: What is currently known? In B. S.McCrady & W. R.Miller (Eds.), *Research on Alcoholics Anonymous: Opportunities and alternatives* (pp. 41–77). New Brunswick, NJ: Rutgers Center for Alcohol Studies.

Flynn, A. M., Alvarez, J., Jason, L. A., Olson, B. D., Ferrari, J. R., & Davis, M. I. (2006). African American Oxford Houses residents: Sources of abstinent social networks. *Journal of Prevention and Intervention in the Community, 31,* 111–119.

Humphreys, K. (2004). *Circles of recovery: Self-help organizations for addictions.* Cambridge, UK: Cambridge University Press.

Jason, L. A., Davis, M. I., Ferrari, J. R., & Bishop, P. D. (2001). Oxford House: A review of research and implications for substance abuse recovery and community research. *Journal of Drug Education, 31,* 1–27.

Jason, L. A., Davis, M. I., Ferrari, J. R., & Anderson, E. (2007). The need for substance abuse after-care: A longitudinal analysis of Oxford House. *Addictive Behaviors, 32,* 803–818

Jason, L. A., Olson, B. D., Ferrari, J. R., & Lo Sasso, A. T. (2006). Communal housing settings enhance substance abuse recovery. *American Journal of Public Health, 91,* 1727–1729.

Kownacki, R. J., & Shadish, W. R. (1999). Does Alcoholics Anonymous work? The results from a meta-analysis of controlled experiments. *Substance Use and Misuse, 34,* 1897–1916.

Kurtz, E. (1979). *Not-God: A History of Alcoholics Anonymous.* Center City, MN: Hazelden.

Longabaugh, R., Wirtz, P. W., Zweben, A., & Stout, R. L. (1998). Network support for drinking, Alcoholics Anonymous and long-term matching effects. *Addiction, 93,* 1313–1333.

Majer, J. M., Jason, L. A., Ferrari, J. R., North, C. S. (2002). Comorbidity among Oxford House residents: A preliminary outcome study. *Addictive Behaviors, 27,* 837–845

Majer, J. M., Jason, L. A., Ferrari, J. R., Venable, L. B., & Olson, B. D. (2002). Social support and self-efficacy for abstinence: Is peer identification an issue? *Journal of Substance Abuse Treatment, 23,* 209–215.

McLellan, A. T., Kushner, H., Metzger, D., Peters, R., Smith, I., Grissom, G., et al. (1992). The fifth edition of the Addiction Severity Index. *Journal of Substance Abuse Treatment, 9,* 199–213.

McCrady, B. S., & Miller, W. R. (1993). *Research on Alcoholics Anonymous: Opportunities and alternatives.* New Brunswick, NJ: Rutgers Center of Alcohol Studies.

Miller, W. R., & Del Boca, F. K. (1994). Measurement of drinking behavior using the Form 90 family of instruments. *Journal of Studies on Alcohol, 12*(Suppl.), 112–118.

Montgomery, H. A., Miller, W. R., & Tonigan, J. S. (1995). Does Alcoholics Anonymous involvement predict treatment outcome? *Journal of Substance Abuse Treatment, 12*, 241–246.

Nealon-Woods, M. A., Ferrari, J. R., & Jason, L. A. (1995). Twelve step program use among Oxford House residents: Spirituality or social support in sobriety? *Journal of Sobstance Abuse, 7*, 311–318.

Oxford House. (2002). *Oxford House manual.* Silver Spring, MD: .

Ouimette, P. C., Moos, R. H., & Finney, J. W. (1998). Influence of outpatient treatment and 12-step group involvement on one-year substance abuse treatment outcomes. *Journal of Studies on Alcohol, 59*, 513–522.

Pisani, V. D., Fawcett, J., Clark, D. C., & McGuire, M. (1993). The relative contributions of medication adherence and AA meeting attendance to abstinent outcome for chronic alcoholics. *Journal of Studies on Alcohol, 54*, 115–119.

Snow, M. G., Prochaska, J. O., & Rossi, J. (1994). Process of Change in Alcoholics Anonymous: Maintenance factors in long-term sobriety. *Journal of Studies on Alcohol, 55*, 362–371.

Tonigan, J. S., Toscova, R., & Miller, W. R. (1996). Meta-analysis of the Alcoholics Anonymous literature: Sample and study characteristics moderate findings. *Journal of Studies on Alcohol, 57*, 65–72.

Wallace, J., McNeill, D., Gilfillan, D., MacLean, K., & Fanella, F. (1988). Six month treatment outcomes in socially stable alcoholics: Abstinence rates. *Journal of Substance Abuse Treatment, 5*, 237–252.

Weisner, C., Greenfield, T., & Room, R. (1995). Trends in the treatment of alcohol problems in the U.S. general population, 1979 through 1990. *American Journal of Public Health, 85*, 55–60.

The Role of Self-Regulation in Abstinence Maintenance: Effects of Communal Living on Self-Regulation

JOSEPH R. FERRARI, PhD, EDWARD B. STEVENS, MBA,
and LEONARD A. JASON, PhD

DePaul University

Studies of self-regulation suggested that self-control requires finite resources; this requirement, in turn, may present a significant challenge for those trying to recover from or control addictive behaviors. The present study examined the relationships between self-regulation and abstinence maintenance among adults in recovery (n = 606: 407 men, 199 women; M age = 38.5 years) residing in self-governed, communal-living, abstinent homes across the United States. Self-regulation scores (controlling for sex and age) were positively related to length of abstinence. In addition, a factor analysis of self-regulation scores resulted in some differentiation between general self-discipline and impulsivity in self-control related to addiction. The relationship between impulsivity and length of abstinence was stronger than the relationship derived between general self-regulation and length of abstinence.

Research on *self-regulation ability* suggested a number of important properties characteristic of an individual's ability to control their behavior. For instance, the greater a person's self-regulation resources the greater likelihood for maintaining a successful lifestyle that person will experience (Tangney, Baumeister, & Boone, 2004). High self-control has been correlated

The authors express gratitude to Meg Davis for supervising data collection and to Josefina Alvarez for advice on data analysis. Funding for this study was made possible in part through National Institute on Drug Abuse (NIDA) grants #5F31DA16037 and # R01DA13231.

with better academic performance (Tangney et al., 2004), mastery at cognitively challenging tasks (Muraven, Tice, & Baumeister, 1998), and the capacity to control aggression (DeWall, Baumeister, Stillman, & Gailliot, 2007). Higher self-regulation scores also correlated with lower likelihood to overeat (Tangney et al., 2004) and greater resistance toward drinking alcoholic beverages (Muraven, Collins, & Nienhaus, 2002). Furthermore, individuals who reported strong self-control claimed better adjustment and fewer reports of psychological distress (Tangney et al. 2004). This depletion effect has been described as comparable to "muscle fatigue" (Muraven & Baumeister, 2000). Thus, self-regulation has dynamic properties related to capacity, usage, and replenishment (Muraven, Shmueli, & Burkley, 2006).

Self-regulation is characterized by behavior consequences suggesting it operates as a finite but renewable resource supporting a significant relationship between strength of self-regulation and beneficial behaviors. The utilization of the self-regulation resource has been tested with the effects of social exclusion, self-presentation (Vohs, Baumeister, & Ciarocco, 2005), intellectual performance, and decision making (Ferrari & Pychyl, 2007). These studies demonstrate the breadth of self-regulation's association across multiple domains of an individual's social well-being. Overall, these studies found that cognitively challenging tasks required discipline that may tax one's self-regulatory resource.

It should be noted that much of the previous research on self-regulation used college students as participants. Little is known how adult men and women, who may experience difficulties in life to regulate their desires, such as persons in recovery for substance abuse (Muraven et al., 2002), may report changes in self-regulation. The present article examined scores on this measure among a sample of adult individuals who were maintaining abstinence and living in communal housing where abstinence maintenance required self-control and relapse rates were high (Jason, Olson, Ferrari, & Lo Sasso, 2006). Studies focused on resisting temptations to addictive behaviors, such as regarding alcohol (Muraven & Shmueli, 2006) and fattening snacks (Tice, Bratslavsky, & Baumeister, 2001), indicated that after being challenged to resist temptation, individuals on average perform less well on tasks or decision making that taxed analogous cognitive processes.

ADDICTIONS, RECOVERY, AND SELF-REGULATION

Baumeister (2002) discussed a theoretical role for self-regulation failure in impulsive behavior. From the perspective of self-regulation, an individual with addictive behaviors may appear to be an exemplar of self-regulation failure. That is, persons addicted to substances generally share two characteristics that are often cited in addiction theory (Becker & Murphy, 1988)—*impulsive consumption*, behaviors that significantly exceed normal levels, and a *failure to assess future consequences* of their behavior. Research on discount rates (how individuals evaluate current versus future rewards) indicated addicts have almost twice the discount rate of a nonaddict control group (Kirby, Petry, & Bickel, 1999). These results suggest that addicts tend to dismiss future consequences in making current decisions when compared to those without past addictions. In addition, the expected hedonic reward (of using) requires significant self-control to resist consumption. Studies on risky gambling choices using a control group, a group of substance-dependent individuals, and a group of individuals with ventromedial lesions resulted in the substance-dependent individuals performing midway between the control group and those with ventromedial lesions (Bechara, Dolan, & Hindes, 2002; Bechara & Damasio, 2002). Those participants with ventromedial lesions went for greater but riskier payoffs, and showed no responsiveness to future consequences. The control group learned a balanced strategy that resulted in near optimal payoffs. Substance-dependent individuals were biased most strongly with an anticipation of a large, current reward, thereby overvaluing the current expectation and not weighting future negative consequences as highly as the control group.

These studies evaluating future consequences and assessing current rewards were consistent with the nature of impulsivity (Baumeister, 2002) and impulsive behavior (Tice et al., 2001). Controlling impulses means resisting short-term rewards or pleasures in order to achieve longer-term goals. Impulsive behavior may result from goal conflict (current pleasure versus goals), lack of self-monitoring (an accurate assessment of current benefits and future consequences), and inadequate self-regulation resources (Baumeister, 2002). These conditions are descriptive of an addict inaccurately assessing both the hedonic pleasure of current usage of an addictive substance and the objective longer term consequences. This multidimensional nature of impulsivity in abstinent alcoholics (*disinhibition* and *discounting*) was also investigated by Dom, De Wilde, Hulstijn, and Sabbe (2006). Similar findings have been found in other impulsivity measures with substance-dependent populations (Dawe, Gullo, & Loxton, 2004). Impulsivity may be considered a common process underlying substance abuse and other behavioral disorders, has been researched as well (Bornovalova, Lejuez, Daughters, Rosenthal, & Lynch, 2005). These studies suggested a strong link between impulsivity and addictive behaviors.

The present study examined impulsivity by trying to separate general qualities of self-discipline from those more closely related to impulsivity. Tangney et al. (2004) found by factor analysis that the full version of self-regulation reduced to five factors; those generally related to self-discipline, resistance to impulsivity, healthy habits, work ethic, and reliability. Because of the stability of the correlations between the factors, Tangney et al. (2004) utilized a self-report measure to tap these five domains. However, in the present study our participant sample consisted of individuals who previously abused substances and were now seeking to maintain abstinence. We investigated the dimension of impulse control explicitly and were interested in whether the Tangney et al. (2004) self-regulation measure captured the dimension of impulsivity when scored by a relatively large sample of adults with histories of substance abuse. Based on prior research of self-regulation (e.g., Muraven, Baumeister, & Tice, 1999; Muraven & Shmueli, 2006), we expected a positive association between self-regulation and length of abstinence. Also, we expected a component of self-regulation, resistance to impulsivity, would be positively associated with length of abstinence.

METHOD

Participants

A total of 606 adult residents (407 men, 199 women) living in one of 170 communal-living settings across the United States called Oxford Houses served as participants in the present study. These participants were part of a larger, longitudinal Oxford House study who participated in the second wave of data collection (Jason, Davis, Ferrari, & Anderson, 2007). At present, there are more than 1,200 Oxford Houses operating across the United States. Each Oxford House is a communal residence that is a rented, single-family house for people recovering from substance abuse (Ferrari, Jason, Sasser, Davis, & Olson, 2006). The houses are resident funded and democratically governed, without restrictions on length of stay, and they operate with minimal rules other than economic sufficiency and a zero tolerance for substance usage (Ferrari, Jason, Davis, Olson, & Alvarez, 2004). Permission to do this study was granted by the DePaul Institutional Review Board.

Participants' mean age was 38.5 years ($SD = 9.4$). Most respondents were Caucasian (59.7%) or African American (31.4%) and single (51.5%) or divorced (29.5%), and they reported on average 12.6 years of education ($SD = 2.1$). Time in residence at an Oxford House averaged 11.7 months ($SD = 15.7$), while average time since last alcohol use averaged 1.7 years ($SD = 2.8$) and drug use was 2.0 years ($SD = 3.0$). Respondents averaged 2.6 ($SD = 4.0$) and 2.8 ($SD = 3.0$) treatment episodes for alcohol and drugs, respectively.

Procedure

Participants were recruited by advertisement in an Oxford House newsletter mailed in 2001 to each house across the United States that existed at the time of the study. In addition, participants were recruited through telephone inquiry to Oxford House presidents in five targeted geographical areas that had the highest density of Oxford Houses (Washington and Oregon, Pennsylvania and New Jersey, North Carolina, Illinois, and Texas). All participants were informed about the purpose, objectives, and methodology of the study and were advised of the voluntary nature of the study before signing and returning a consent form. Each participant then completed the self-report measures of self-regulation, addiction-recovery history, and abstinence maintenance. Upon completion of the surveys, each participant was paid $15. More details about the study methodology can be found in Jason et al. (2007).

Psychometric Measures

All participants completed the Addiction Severity Index—Lite (ASI; McLellan et al., 1992), which assessed common difficulties associated with substance abuse (e.g., drug use, alcohol use, and illegal activity). This instrument has been used extensively over the last 15 years and has demonstrated excellent test–retest reliability ($\geq$0.83; McLellan et al., 1992). Utilizing only subsections of the scale has been deemed appropriate and psychometrically sound by McLellan et al. (1992), and for the present study sociodemographic data and substance abuse history were obtained. Objective questions measured the number, extent, and duration of problem symptoms for both the person's lifetime and within the last 30 days. This instrument also collected information on length of current abstinence period for both drug and alcohol usage. Makela (2004) found high internal consistency for medical status, alcohol, use and psychiatric status, and the ASI has been used successfully in previous outcome studies with Oxford House residents (e.g., Jason et al., 2006; Jason et al., 2007).

Participants also completed the *Alcohol & Substance Abuse—Form 90 Timeline Followback* (Miller & Del Boca, 1994), which collects information regarding general health care utilization, residential history, and alcohol and drug usage over the prior 90 days. Reliability on this instrument was found to be good to excellent for all summary measures of alcohol consumption and illicit drugs that were most frequently used, *retest r* $\geq$ 0.90 for both alcohol usage and drug usage (Tonigan, Miller, & Brown, 1997). This instrument has been used in previously in Oxford House studies (Jason et al., 2007).

Self-regulation was examined by having participants complete the self-regulation scale (Tangney et al., 2004), which consists of 13 items scored on a 5-point Likert scale (1 = *not at all*, 5 = *very much*). Examples of questions include *I do certain things that are bad for me, if they are fun* and *I am able to work effectively toward long-term goals.* Tangney et al. (2004) reported that this measure had good internal consistency (alpha *r* = 0.83 to 0.85), and with the present sample Cronbach's alpha was 0.82 (*M* = 44.1; *SD* = 8.2).

RESULTS

Factor Analysis of Self-Regulation Items

We factored the self-control scale to investigate whether a logical underlying dimension of impulse control could be isolated. Tangney et al. (2004) in

TABLE 1 Factor Loadings for the Tagney et al. (2004) Self-regulation Measure

	Factor 1 General	Factor 2 Impulse
I am good at resisting temptation		.67
I have a hard time breaking bad habits	.45	
I am lazy	.46	
I say inappropriate things	.54	
I do certain things that are bad for me, if they are fun	.51	
I refuse things that are bad for me		.54
I wish I had more discipline	.42	
People would say I have iron discipline		.64
Pleasure and fun sometimes keep me from getting work done	.59	
I have trouble concentrating	.59	
I am able to work effectively toward long-term goals		.49
Sometimes I can't stop myself from doing something, even if I know it's wrong	.48	
I often act without thinking through all the alternatives	.65	
Eigenvalue	2.56	1.91
Percentage of Variance Explained	19.67	14.67

n = 606.

developing this self-control scale used factor analysis and extracted five relevant dimensions (self-discipline, inclination toward nonimpulsive behavior, healthy habits, work ethic, and reliability). Nevertheless, the authors used the scale as a uni-dimensional measure. In the present study, factor analysis extracted dimensions using a *maximum likelihood process with varimax rotation*. A two-factor solution, shown in Table 1, accounted for 34.3% of the total variance and was statistically significant, $\chi^2 (53) = 201.5, p <.001$. The relatively low explanation of variance results from the items of this scale mostly being weakly positively correlated overall (*interclass r* = 0.224, *mode* = 0.110, *range* = 0.010 to 0.460); thus these questions were mostly additive to the overall scale and provided unique contributions to the overall variance. The between factors correlation was $r = 0.149$. Although the total variance explained by the factor analysis was less than optimal, the prior findings (Tangney et al., 2004), statistical significance, and average unique variance of the individual questions in the instrument made the exploratory use of the factor results acceptable.

Nine of the thirteen questions made up the first factor. This factor, called *general self-discipline*, focused more on general patterns of behavior. For example, questions included *I am lazy* and *I have trouble concentrating*. The reliability of this scale was good, with a Cronbach's alpha = 0.80 (*M* = 31.1. *SD* = 6.25). The second factor, labeled *impulse control*, consisted of the remaining four questions (e.g., *I am good at resisting temptation* and *I am able to work effectively toward long-term goals*). This measure had a Cronbach's alpha = 0.69 (*M* = 12.9. *SD* = 3.27).

Multiple Regression Analysis

To test the relationship between the self-regulation factors and time abstinent, a multiple regression was performed that controlled for the demographic variables of sex and age. Sex and age were demographic variables that were significant covariates with time abstinent but not the self-regulation factors. Time abstinent was normalized using a natural log transformation to preserve rank order and achieve a normal distribution of reported durations of abstinence. The independent variables consisted of *general self-discipline* and *impulse control*. The resulting model was significant, $R^2 = .131$, $F(4,601) = 22.594$, $p < .001$. With respect to the standardized coefficients for the self-regulation factors, the general self-discipline factor was insignificant, $\beta = -.007$, $t(601) = -.172$, $p = .863$. The factor associated with resisting temptation was significant, $\beta = .164$, $t(604) = 4.246$, $p < .001$. These results supported the expectation that resistance to impulsive behaviors would be positively related to abstinence time.

A second regression tested the overall self-regulation measure with time abstinent. The model was significant with $R^2 = .114$, $F(3,602) = 25.777$, $p < .001$. The standardized coefficient for the self-regulation score was $\beta = .10$, $t(603) = 2.522$, $p < .05$. Thus, the impulse control score was a better predictor for time abstinent in this sample than the overall self-regulation measure, $\beta_{impulse} = .164 > \beta_{general} = .100$. Overall, the results of this analysis supported the positive relationship between self-regulation and time abstinent. Additionally, the investigation into a relationship between an impulsivity control and time abstinent was supportive of a positive relationship.

DISCUSSION

For our sample of Oxford House residents, this cross-sectional analysis suggested that resistance to impulsivity, as well as overall self-regulation strength, had a positive relationship with time abstinence. These results supported the predictions that self-regulation was positively related to time abstinent, and, more specifically, that impulsivity control would have a greater positive association with abstinence. While the average effect sizes were small, these findings are consistent with previous addiction research (Dom et al., 2006) and research on self-regulation (Tice et al., 2001; Muraven & Shmueli, 2006).

This study benefited from utilizing as participants a sample of Oxford House residents who were maintaining abstinence. These individuals provided self-report measures of abstinence and self-regulation. Both the general self-control measure and impulsivity resistance factor were significant. The impulsivity resistance factor alone was derived from factoring a scale that was largely additive in nature; thus the proportion of overall variance explained by factoring was less than typically found. Further investigation of impulsivity control and abstinence might benefit our understanding of longitudinal changes of self-regulation during recovery and provide improvements in measures of the concept among adult samples.

Limitations and Future Directions

Limitations of the study include a cross-sectional design, and the total variance explained by the factor analysis was less than optimal. The findings of the present study, despite limitations, may provide a basis for further study in self-regulation, impulsivity, and behaviors related to addiction and abstinence. For instance, an understanding of the dynamics of self-regulation and abstinence maintenance over time might provide an insight on the usage and replenishment of self-regulation resources (Muraven & Baumeister, 2000). This finding might possibly include inclusion of more multidimensional measures of impulsivity control as suggested by Dom et al. (2007) and Dawe et al. (2004).

Another possible path of investigation would be to examine associated behaviors of addiction (e.g., criminal activity, employment stability) with self-regulation and impulsivity to better understand these relationships. Self-regulation has been investigated across a variety of domains (Tangney et al., 2004) including aggression (Wall et al., 2007) with significant results. The relationship between self-regulation, impulsivity, and addictive and related behaviors might be significant and predictive. Because all participants in the present study were Oxford House residents, future research might focus on the measurement of self-regulation, impulsivity, and abstinent behavior of individuals residing in other recovery treatment living arrangements. Research between housing condition groups might provide some insight into the relationships between residential arrangements and self-regulation.

In short, the present study suggested that self-regulation in general and resistance to impulsivity, more specifically, were positively related to time abstinent in a cross-sectional study of recovering substance dependent participants who resided in Oxford Houses, a communal living arrangement supporting abstinence. Continued research on these relationships might include longitudinal investigations, research of other related addictive behaviors, introduction of varied measures, and different adult samples. These findings have implications for group work because they suggest that self-regulation is an important goal for therapists and that a variety of group interventions might be helpful in fostering this domain.

REFERENCES

Baumeister, R. F. (2002). Yielding to temptation: Self-control failure, impulsive purchasing, and consumer behavior. *Journal of Consumer Research, 28,* 670–676

Bechara, A., & Damasio, H. (2002). Decision-making and addiction, Part I: Impaired activation of somatic states in substance dependent individuals when pondering decisions with negative future consequences. *Neuropsychologia, 40,* 1675–1689.

Bechara, A., Dolan, S., & Hindes, A. (2002). Decision-making and addiction, Part II: Myopia for the future or hypersensitivity to reward? *Neuropsychologia, 40,* 1690–1705.

Becker, G. S., & Murphy, K. M. (1988). A theory of rational addiction. *Journal of Political Economy, 96,* 675–700.

Bornovalova, M. A., Lejuez, C. W., Daughters, S. B., Rosenthal, M. Z., & Lynch, T. R. (2005). Impulsivity as a common process across borderline personality and substance use disorders. *Clinical Psychology Review, 25,* 790–812

Dawe, S., Gullow, M. J., & Loxton, N. J. (2004). Reward drive and rash impulsiveness as dimensions of impulsivity: Implications for substance abuse. *Addictive Behaviors, 29,* 1389–1405

Dom, G., De Wilde, B., Hulstijn, W., & Sabbe, B. (2007). Dimensions of impulsive behaviour in abstinent alcoholics. *Personality and Individual Differences, 42*(3), 465–476.

Ferrari, J. R., Jason, L. A., Sasser, K. C., Davis, M. I., & Olson, B. D. (2006). Creating a home to promote recovery: The physical environments of Oxford House. *Journal of Prevention & Intervention in the Community, 31,* 27–40

Ferrari, J. R., Jason, L. A., Davis, M. I., Olson, B. D., & Alvarez, J. (2004). Similarities and differences in governance among residents in drug and/or alcohol misuse: Self vs. staff rules and regulations. *Therapeutic Communities: The International Journal for Therapeutic and Supportive Organizations, 25,* 179–192.

Ferrari, J. R., & Pychyl, T. A. (2007). Regulating speed, accuracy, and judgments by indecisives: Effects of frequent choices on self-regulation failure. *Personality and Individual Differences, 42,* 777–782.

Jason, L. A., Olson, B. D., Ferrari, J. R., Lo Sasso, A. T. (2006). Communal housing settings enhance substance abuse recovery. *American Journal of Public Health, 96,* 1727–1729

Jason, L. A., Davis, M. I., Ferrari, J. R., & Anderson, E. (2007). The need for substance abuse after-care: A longitudinal analysis of Oxford House. *Addictive Behaviors, 32,* 803–818

Kirby, K. N., Petry, N. M., and Bickel, W. K. (1999). Heroin addicts have higher discount rates for delayed rewards than non-drug-using controls. *Journal of Experimental Psychology: General, 128,* 78–87.

Makela, K. (2004). Studies of the reliability and validity of the Addiction Severity Index. *Addiction, 99,* 398–410.

McLellan, A. T., Kushner, H., Metzger, D., Peters, R., Smith, I., Grissom, G., et al. (1992). The fifth edition of the Addiction Severity Index. *Journal of Substance Abuse Treatment, 9,* 199–213.

Miller, W. R., & Del Boca, F. K. (1994). Measurement of drinking behavior using the Form 90 family of instruments. *Journal of Studies on Alcohol, 12*(Suppl.), 112–118.

Muraven, M., & Baumeister, R. F. (2000). Self-regulation and depletion of limited resources: Does self-control resemble a muscle? *Psychological Bulletin, 126,* 247–259.

Muraven, M., Baumeister, R. F., & Tice, D. M. (1999). Longitudinal improvement of self-regulation through practice: Building self-control strength through repeated exercise. *Journal of Social Psychology, 139,* 446–457.

Muraven, M., Collins, R. L., & Nienhaus, K. (2002). Self-control and alcohol restraint: An initial application of the self-control strength model. *Psychology of Addictive Behaviors, 16,* 113–120.

Muraven, M., & Shmueli, D. (2006). The self-control costs of fighting the temptation to drink. *Psychology of Addictive Behaviors, 20,* 154–160.

Muraven, M., Shmueli, D., & Burkley, E. (2006). Conserving self-control strength. *Journal of Personality and Social Psychology, 91,* 524–537.

Muraven, M., Tice, D. M., & Baumeister, R. F. (1998). Self-control as a limited resource: Regulatory depletion patterns. *Journal of Personality and Social Psychology, 74*(3), 774–789.

Tangney, J. P., Baumeister, R. F., & Boone, A. L. (2004). High self-control predicts good adjustment, less pathology, better grades, and interpersonal success. *Journal of Personality, 72,* 271–322.

Tice, D. M., Bratslavsky, E., & Baumeister, R. F. (2001). Emotional distress regulation takes precedence over impulse control: If you feel bad, do it! *Journal of Personality and Social Psychology, 80,* 53–67.

Tonigan, J. S., Miller, W. R., and Brown, J. M. (1997). The reliability of Form 90: An instrument for assessing alcohol treatment outcome. *Journal for Studies of Alcohol, 58,* 358–364.

Vohs, K. D., Baumeister, R. F., & Ciarocco, N. J. (2005). Self-regulation and self-presentation: Regulatory resource depletion impairs impression management and effortful self-presentation depletes regulatory resources. *Journal of Personality and Social Psychology, 88,* 632–657.

Hope and Substance Abuse Recovery: The Impact of Agency and Pathways within an Abstinent Communal-Living Setting

GLEN M. MATHIS, MA, JOSEPH R. FERRARI, PhD,
DAVID R. GROH, PhD, and LEONARD A. JASON, PhD

DePaul University

Hope is commonly divided into two constructs: agency, defined as goal-directed energy, and pathways, defined as the ability to create paths to a goal. To date, only two studies have examined the utility of hope in substance abuse recovery, and the present investigation builds on this small literature by assessing hope beliefs within a larger and more diverse sample of adults in recovery. This study examined how two hope constructs of agency and pathways related to substance use abstinence among 90 new residents of communal-living recovery homes (i.e., Oxford Houses) who completed two waves of data assessment. Results indicated that agency scores significantly predicted alcohol use at Wave 1, but pathway scores failed to predict drug or alcohol use at this time point. Additionally, agency and pathway scores predicted drug (but not alcohol use) at an 8-month follow-up assessment. These findings indicated that participants' hope may be linked to substance use at later stages of recovery. In addition, these results suggested a stronger relationship between hope and drug as opposed to alcohol use at this time point. Implications for substance abuse recovery are discussed.

The concept of hope became popular with psychologists in the late twentieth century (Lopez, Snyder, & Teramoto, 2003). Since then, hope has

---

Portions of this article were based on a master's thesis by the first author under the direction of the second author. Funding was made possible in part through National Institute on Drug Abuse grants #5F31DA16037 and # R01DA13231.

been conceptualized in a variety of ways. To start out with, hope can be viewed as a *dispositional* or a *state* construct. *Dispositional* measures of hope view hope as a long-term trait, whereas *state* measures of hope conceptualize hope as a short-term, temporary construct. Although state and trait measures may differ conceptually, an individual's score on measures of dispositional and state hope do not vary greatly, as state hope typically fluctuates within a limited range around a person's level of dispositional hope (Snyder, Sympson, Ybasco, Borders, Babyak, & Higgins, 1996).

In addition, most theories of hope fall into two categories: *emotion*-based or *cognition*-based (Snyder, Harris, Anderson, Holleran, Irving, & Sigmon, 1991). Of the few *emotion*-based hope theories that exist, most of these include some sort of cognitive element (Lopez et al., 2003). Beginning with Mowrer (1960), hope was an emotional form of secondary reinforcement. More recently, Averill, Catlin, and Chon (1990) described hope as an emotion governed by cognition. In their model, individuals were most likely to experience hope when they possessed goals that were realistically within their reach, personally important to them, and socially and morally acceptable (Averill et al.).

In contrast to the emotion-based models, the models based on *cognition* receive much more attention by researchers (Lopez et al., 2003). For example, Godfrey (1987) viewed hope as the belief in the possibility of a pleasant outcome. In Gottschalk's (1974) theory, hope was defined by positive expectancy or the level of confidence that a particular pleasurable outcome was likely to occur. Furthermore, according to Erikson's (1964) theory of hope, hope is part of healthy cognitive development and is defined as an enduring belief in the attainability of primal wishes in spite of the anarchic urges and rages of dependency (Erikson). Finally, Staats's (1989) theory of hope combined Erikson's model with expectancy theories and posited that hope is the relationship between wishes and expectations. Hope is a mediator that calculates expectations of success and the emotional intensity of the wish or desire.

Currently, the most accepted model of hope considered the construct to be much more complex (Snyder, 1994; Snyder et al., 1991). Snyder's model consisted of three interrelated cognitive components, identified as *goals*, *agency*, and *pathways* (Snyder, Ilardi, Michael, & Cheavens, 2000). This hope theory assumed that human actions were *goal-oriented*, and that goals were targets of mental action sequences (Snyder et al., 2000). Snyder (1994) proposed that goals must be sufficiently important to motivate people and that unclear goals do not provide the mental spark for adequate motivation (Snyder, LaPointe, Crowson, & Early, 1998; Snyder, 1994). Also, goals that motivate people should be within reach and contain some inherent uncertainty. Finally, goals do not have a time restraint and may vary from short to long term (Irving, Snyder, Cheavens, Gravel, Hanke, & Hillberg, 2004).

Agency was a sense of goal-directed energy and determination in meeting one's goals (Snyder et al., 1991). It was a mental energy that pushed a person toward the goal and a driving force in hopeful thinking (Snyder, 1994). Agency was the willpower and commitment that enabled people to pursue and maintain a goal they were attending at any given moment. Some examples of agency thoughts were "I know I can do this," "I've got what it takes," and "I will get this done." *Pathway* was an ability to create alternate routes or paths to the goal, especially when a goal was hindered (Snyder et al., 1991). To initiate an imagined goal, people believed that they were competent of producing practical routes to the goal or generating alternate paths when the original fails (Irving et al., 2004). People with high levels of pathway thinking often perceive that they can come up with multiple ways to attain their goals (Snyder et al., 1991).

Although agency and pathway thinking were associated, each represents a distinct construct (Babyak, Snyder, & Yoshinobu, 1993; Snyder et al., 1996). Therefore, the popular expression "Where there is a will there is a way" is not wholly accurate. People who possessed a successful sense of agency ("the will") may or may not perceive the pathways ("the way") to their goals (Snyder et al., 1991). One may possess the motivation (agency) to complete a goal, but be unable to see clearly the route to accomplish the goal (pathways). Alternatively, one may see many routes to a goal (pathways) without possessing drive to accomplish the goal (agency). To successfully obtain goals in one's life, both a sense of agency and pathway must be present (Snyder et al., 1991, 1996).

THE ROLE OF HOPE IN SUBSTANCE ABUSE RECOVERY

A hopeful style of thinking was associated with adaptive coping and greater adjustment in the face of stress (Snyder, 1994; Snyder et al., 1996). Substance abusers in treatment may attempt to reach the challenging goal of long-term abstinence but must remain highly determined to the process of recovery (Irving, Seinder, Burling, Pagliarini, & Robbins-Sisco, 1998). Hope may be an important component of recovery from substance abuse, a goal that must be pursued with incredible willpower given repeated challenges (Marlatt, 1998). Persons who perceive recovery as attainable and within their control may remain more committed to recovery over time despite repeated challenges to that goal (Irving et al.).

Individuals who pursue recovery from substance abuse must be prepared to generate pathways as strategies to cope with obstacles and skills to handle "triggers" that may lead to relapse (Marlatt, 1998). People with strong hope beliefs were well prepared to deal with situational threats, were able to generate a greater number of strategies for attaining goals (Snyder et al., 1991), and increased their commitment to appropriate adaptive strategies in the face of threats (Irving et al., 1998). Persons with strong hope beliefs may be more adept at generating and implementing strategies to prevent relapse and resuming their commitment to recovery following a relapse.

Currently, only two studies investigated the utility of hope in the area of substance abuse recovery. Jackson, Wernicke, and Haaga (2003) examined dispositional (trait) hope as a predictor of entering a voluntary substance abuse treatment program for federal prison inmates ($n = 1001$). Contrary to predictions, increased hope was actually associated with a lower probability of entering treatment. Jackson et al. argued that in the context of incarceration and substance abuse, high levels of hope may indicate excessive self-reliance and an underestimated need for professional treatment. In the second study, Irving et al. (1998) examined the relationship between state (current) hopeful thinking about goals and recovery from substance abuse among residents and graduates of a residential treatment program for substance-dependent homeless veterans ($n = 90$). As predicted, higher state hope was related to longer lengths of abstinence. Unfortunately, the study of Irving et al. was limited by a small sample lacking in diversity. The present investigation extends that project by assessing hope beliefs within a larger and more diverse sample of adults in recovery. As done by Jackson and colleagues, the current study investigated the relationship between dispositional hope and substance abuse recovery.

The current study used a sample of adults residing in one of a national network of *Oxford Houses (OH)*, a substance abuse recovery program that applied principles of supportive mutual help to addiction treatment (Ferrari, Jason, Olson, Davis, & Alvarez, 2002; Jason, Davis, Ferrari, & Bishop, 2001). Each communal-living setting was a rented, multiroom dwelling for same-sex occupants, located in low-crime areas and operated democratically by majority rule by occupants electing house officers every 6 months (see Jason, Ferrari, Davis, & Olson, 2006, for details). Presently, there are over 1,200 dwellings throughout the USA (Jason et al., 2007).

In summary, because substance abuse is such a devastating affliction, any further knowledge about specific traits that may increase the chances of a successful recovery would be greatly beneficial to the field. Dispositional hope may be a useful mechanism for understanding the common process in psychological change (Snyder et al., 1998). Hopeful thinking might relate to success in achieving goals and might relate to successful recovery from substance abuse. Irving et al. (1998) suggested that levels of hope may positively relate to substance abuse recovery. Because the hope theory of Snyder et al. (1991) focused on a goal-oriented process, and because attaining long-term substance abuse abstinence is tremendously challenging, it was hypothesized in the present study that dispositional levels of hope would positively predict abstinence.

METHOD

Participants

The data analyzed for the present study were based on participants in a larger national study on Oxford House who completed self-report measures at baseline and again 8 months later. Initially, the sample consisted of 897 current OH residents (292 women, 604 men). Of this sample, 588 participants also completed the second 8-month measurement wave, indicating a 65.55% retention rate. In order to control for the fact that participants had varied lengths of stay in OH at baseline, we only included participants who lived in a house for a month or less at baseline 'and who were retained 8 months later ($n = 96$). The average age of this sample was 35.5 years ($SD = 8.2$), and the average education level was 12.5 years ($SD = 1.8$). The majority of the sample was European American (58.3%), single/never married (55.3%), and employed full-time (64.6%), with an average monthly income of $630.4 ($SD = 706.6$). Participants on average had used alcohol for 16.3 years (SD = 9.5), and the illicit drugs of choice within this sample included cannabis (average of 9.8 years, $SD = 9.6$) and cocaine (average of 7.9 years, $SD = 7.7$), among others. Finally, participants on average were poly-substance users for 9.7 years ($SD = 9.4$).

Procedure

Participants were recruited and surveyed using two strategies. Most participants (88.9%) were recruited by an announcement published in the monthly OH newsletter distributed to all of the established Oxford Houses. Other individuals filled out baseline questionnaires at an annual OH convention. Analyses of data collected by these two methods did not reveal significant differences in outcome variables. For all participants, staff members explained that participation was entirely voluntary and confidential, and withdrawal without consequence was possible at any time. In addition, participants filled out a telephone contact sheet for future waves of data collection. The length of completing these measures was on average >90 minutes. For the 8-month follow-up wave, research staff contacted participants based on the telephone contact sheet. Once contacted, surveys were administered in person, via phone, or by mail. After completing each wave of data collection, participants were given a check for $15. This investigation was approved by an institutional review board.

Measures

Demographic information was obtained from the fifth edition of the Addiction Severity Index—Lite (ASI; McLellan, Kushner, Metzger, Peters, Smith,

Grissom et al., 1992), which has been used extensively in substance abuse studies over the past 15 years and has excellent test–retest reliability ($r >$ 0.83; McLellan et al., 1992). The ASI assessed common problems related to substance abuse: medical status, drug use, alcohol use, illegal activity, family relations, and psychiatric condition. In addition, questions in the ASI measured the number, extent, and duration of problem symptoms in the person's lifetime and in the past 30 days. For the present study, pertinent demographic and background information included age, sex, ethnicity, years of drug use, and whether participants abused alcohol, drugs, or both alcohol and drugs.

Participants also completed Miller and Del Boca's (1994) Form 90 *Timeline Follow-Back*, which measured general health care utilization, residential history, and past 90 days' alcohol and drug use. Form 90 has good reliability for all key summary measures of alcohol consumption, psychosocial functioning, and frequently used illicit drugs. The alcohol and drug use outcomes were assessed using items from this measure: *90 days consumed any amount of alcohol* and *number of days using [type of substance] in past 90 days* (Miller & Del Boca, 1994).

Finally, participants completed the 12-item Adult Dispositional Hope Scale (Snyder et al., 1991), a goal-oriented measure of dispositional or trait-like hope including *agency* thinking (4 items: *I energetically pursue my goals*; alpha $= 0.71$ to 0.76; M score $= 22.01$) and *pathways* thinking (4 items: *I can think of many ways to get out of a jam; M* score $= 23.79$; Cronbach's alpha $= 0.63$ to 0.80). The scale has shown internal consistency within and across factors (Babyak et al., 1993) along with good test–retest reliability over a 10-week period (Cronbach's alpha $= 0.82$; Snyder et al.), suggesting that the construct being measured is truly dispositional in nature, as opposed to state. Each item is rated along an 8-point Likert Scale (1 $=$ *definitely false*: 8 $=$ *definitely true*), with scores ranging from 8 to 64.

RESULTS

Linear regressions explored the relationship between dispositional hope scores and responses on drug and alcohol use in the past 90 days. Although agency scores significantly predicted reported alcohol abstinence at baseline, $\beta = -.25$, t (94) $= 3.69$, $p < .05$, the remaining linear regressions at the same wave were not significant (see Table 1). As evident in Table 2, hope scores predicted substance abstinence at the 8-month follow-up, with agency scores, $\beta = -.35$, t (94) $= 4.18$, $p < .001$, and pathway scores. $\beta = -.34$, t (94) $= 4.00$, $p < .001$. Finally, *zero-order correlates* between hope scores and key demographic characteristics (gender, age, race or ethnicity, marital status, religious preference, years of education, employment status, length of sobriety, and length of stay in Oxford House) were not significant,

TABLE 1 Summary of Regression Analysis for Predicting Substance Abuse Recovery from Agency and Pathway Scores at Baseline

	B	SE B	ß
Predicting agency scores:			
90-day alcohol use	−.77	.31	−.25*
90-day drug use	−.03	.56	−.01
Predicting pathway scores:			
90-day alcohol use	−.26	.38	−.07
90-day drug use	−.14	.66	−.02

$n = 96$.
*$p < .05$.
Note. Negative beta weights indicate greater abstinence.

suggesting that the relationship between hope and substance abstinence was not driven by these types of variables.

DISCUSSION

The current study examined how dispositional hope, reflected by both agency (goal-directed energy and determination) and pathway (ability to create routes or paths to a goal), related to drug and alcohol abstinence within a sample of adults residing in substance abuse recovery homes. It was expected that dispositional hope scores would predict positive substance abuse recovery, with "recovery" operationalized as the number of days abstinent. In order to investigate the ability of the hope beliefs to significantly predict substance abuse recovery, *linear regressions* were run at both measurement waves from a larger study of Oxford House (Jason et al., 2007). Agency scores significantly predicted reported alcohol abstinence at baseline. At an 8-month follow-up, agency and pathway scores predicted reported drug but not alcohol abstinence.

TABLE 2 Summary of Regression Analysis Predicting Substance Abuse Recovery from Agency and Pathway Scores at Follow-up

	B	SE B	ß
Predicting agency scores:			
90-day alcohol use	−.30	.23	−.14
90-day drug use	−.90	.25	−.35***
Predicting pathway scores:			
90-day alcohol use	−.43	.25	−.18
90-day drug use	−.97	.27	−.34***

$n = 96$.
***$p < .001$.
Note. Negative beta weights indicate greater abstinence.

Since all participants were new residents of this communal-living recovery program, these findings indicate that hope predicted substance abstinence at later stages of recovery. In addition, these results indicate a stronger relationship between hope and drug as opposed to alcohol use after an extended period of residence in a totally substance-free setting. While our predictions were partially supported, results may be because participants were less likely to report drug than alcohol use. There are often harsh legal ramifications for being caught with drugs, and little to no legal ramifications for being caught with alcohol. Still, substance abuse is such a major problem in the United States that increased knowledge on successful recovery seems important for clinicians treating people with substance abuse. Individuals entering substance abuse treatment programs with weak hopefulness beliefs may need to be closely monitored and supported, as they are prone to relapse.

Regarding limitations, the current study's sample of Oxford House residents were required to be sober upon entry into the program; therefore, they might have been further along in their recovery compared to individuals in other treatment modalities. In the present study only 67.78% of participants were retained between the first and third waves. Although no differences were found for dispositional hope variables between the continued participants and "drop-outs" at their baseline measurement, it is possible that adults who dropped out had shorter lengths of alcohol and drug sobriety within this communal-living substance-free setting. That limited time within Oxford House might have impacted on their acquisition of strong hope beliefs. Also, all data were self-reports of substance use and abstinence. Because any substance use was grounds for eviction from an Oxford House (Ferrari et al., 2002), it is possible that participants failed to report their actual substance use. Finally, this study only examined dispositional or trait measures of hope within a substance abuse recovery population, and it is suggested that future researchers also examine state or current measures of hope within this population. Nevertheless, the present study suggests that hope beliefs may play a positive and significant role in substance abuse recovery.

REFERENCES

Averill, J. R., Catlin, G., & Chon, K. K. (1990). *Rules of hope*. New York: Springer-Verlag.

Babyak, M. A., Synder, C. R., & Yoshinobu, L. (1993). Psychometric properties of the Hope scale: A confirmatory factor analysis. *Journal of Research in Personality*, *27*, 154–169.

Erickson, E. H. (1964). *Insight and responsibility*. New York: W. W. Norton.

Ferrari, J. R., Jason, L. A., Olson, B. D., Davis, M. I., & Alvarez, J. (2002). Sense of community among Oxford House residents recovering from substance abuse:

Making a house a home. In. A. Fischer (Ed), *Psychological sense of community* (pp. 109–122). New York: Kluwer/Plenum.

Godfrey, J. J. (1987). *A philosophy of human hope*. Dordrecht: Martinus Nijhoff.

Gottschalk, L. (1974). A hope scale applicable to verbal samples. *Archives of General Psychiatry, 30*, 779–785.

Irving, L. M., Seinder, A. L., Burling, T. A., Pagliarini, R., & Robbins-Sisco, D. (1998). Hope and recovery from substance dependence in homeless veterans. *Journal of Social and Clinical Psychology, 17*, 389–406.

Irving, L. M., Snyder, C. R., Cheavens, J., Gravel, L., Hanke, J., & Hilberg, P. (2004). The relationships between hope and outcomes at the pretreatment, beginning, and later phases of psychotherapy. *Journal of Psychotherapy Integration, 14*, 419–443.

Jackson, R., Wernicke, R., & Haaga, D. A. F. (2003). Hope as a predictor of entering substance abuse treatment. *Addictive Behaviors, 28*, 13–28.

Jason, L. A., Davis, M. I., Ferrari, J. R., & Anderson, E. (2007). The need for substance abuse after-care: A longitudinal analysis of Oxford House. *Addictive Behaviors, 32*, 803–818.

Jason, L. A., Davis, M. I., Ferrari, J. R., & Bishop, P. D. (2001). Oxford house: A review of research and implications for substance abuse recovery and community research. *Journal of Drug Education, 31*, 1–27.

Jason, L. A., Davis, M. I., Ferrari, J. R., & Olson, B. D. (2006). *Creating communities for addiction recovery: The Oxford House Model*. Binghamtom, NY: Haworth.

Lopez, S. J., Snyder, C. R., & Teramoto, J. (2003). Hope: Many definitions, many measures. In S. J. Lopez & C. R. Snyder (Eds.), *Positive psychological assessment*. Washington, DC: American Psychological Association.

Marlatt, G. A. (Ed.). (1998). *Harm reduction: Pragmatic strategies for managing high-risk behaviors*. New York: Guildford.

Snyder, C. R. (1994). *The psychology of hope: You can get there from here*. New York: Free Press.

Snyder, C. R., Harris, C., Anderson, J. R., Holleran, S. A., Irving, L. M., & Sigmon, S. T. (1991). The will and the ways: Development and validation of an individual-differences measure of hope. *Journal of Personality and Social Psychology, 60*, 570–585.

Snyder, C. R., Ilardi, S., Michael, S., & Cheavens, J. (2000). Hope theory: Updating a common process for psychological change. In C. R. Snyder & R. E. Ingram (Eds.), *Handbook of psychological change: Psychotherapy processes and practices for the 21st century* (pp. 128–153). New York: Wiley.

Snyder, C. R., LaPointe, A. B., Crowson, J. J., & Early, S. (1998). Preferences of high- and low-hope people for self-referential input. *Cognition and Emotion, 12*, 807–823.

Snyder, C. R., Sympson, S. C., Ybasco, F. C., Borders, T. F., Babyak, M. A., & Higgins, R. L. (1996). Development and validation of the state hope scale. *Journal of Personality and Social Psychology, 70*, 321–335.

Staats, S. (1989). Hope: A comparison of two self-report measures for adults. *Journal of Personality Assessment, 53*, 366–375.

Self-Reports of Substance Abusers: The Impact of Social Desirability on Social Network Variables

DAVID R. GROH, PhD, JOSEPH R. FERRARI, PhD, and
LEONARD A. JASON, PhD

DePaul University

It is important to examine social desirability when interpreting self-report data from substance abusers. Social desirability is the tendency to respond on surveys that make people appear more favorable to others; thus, a strong desire for social approval is related to minimized reports of substance use. In the present study, the relationship between social desirability and different types of social support was examined within 582 residents of communal-living recovery homes (i.e., Oxford Houses). Although effect sizes were small, results may suggest that participants reported social network variables in a socially desirable manner; this tendency toward self-deception even predicted misrepresentations of these constructs 8 months later. In addition, self-reports of the substance use habits of friends and family were more prone to social desirability than the reporting of other social network characteristics. Overall, it is suggested that social desirability might be taken into account when examining substance abusers' self-reports of social support variables.

For individuals in substance abuse recovery, contextual characteristics of the social environment such as social network characteristics may affect treatment acceptance and provide resources that influence posttreatment

Funding was made possible in part through National Institute on Drug Abuse (NIDA) grants #5F31DA16037 and # R01DA13231.

functioning (Finney, Moos, & Mewborn, 1980). Consequently, it is important to explore the social support networks available to people in recovery. Although social support is defined as the resources that other people provide, it is a concept that may be broken down into different dimensions (Cohen, Underwood, & Gottlieb, 2000; Cohen & Wills, 1985; Haber, Cohen, Lucas, & Baltes, 2007).

It may be important to distinguish between *general social support* and *alcohol- or drug-specific support* (Longabaugh & Beattie, 1986). *General social support* is defined as support for the recipient's overall well-being (Cohen et al., 2000; Cohen & Wills, 1985). Measures of general support often combine structural aspects (e.g., the number of people in a network) with functional aspects (e.g., the meaningfulness of that support) to obtain a global assessment of network social support. *Specific social support*, in contrast, may be directly tied to certain functions such as alcohol or illicit drug use (Longabaugh & Beattie). This specific support has either a positive or negative impact on recovery, depending on whether the relationships provide encouragement for abstinence or reduced use (i.e., *specific support for abstinence*) or encouragement for drinking (i.e., *specific support for alcohol or drug use*; Falkin & Strauss, 2003).

Researchers (e.g., Rychtarik, Tarnowski, & St. Lawrence, 1989) argued that social desirability is important to examine when interpreting self-report data from substance abusers (e.g., social network information). *Socially desirable responding* includes the tendency to supply answers on self-report surveys that make a respondent appear more favorable to others than they are in reality (Bradburn, 1983). The prevailing model of social desirability contains two dimensions: *impression management*, the tendency to make purposeful modifications of information to impress others or to avoid negative appraisal, and self-deceptive enhancement, the tendency to believe augmented positive statements about oneself, even if they are not completely accurate (Paulhus, 1984, 1991; Paulhus & Reid, 1991).

A negative relationship has been found between socially desirable responding and reports of substance abuse, and this type of response bias likely results in underestimated rates of use, with heavy users actually reporting less use than light users (Cox, Swinson, Direnfeld, & Bourdeau, 1994; Richards & Pai, 2003). A strong desire for social approval, therefore, may be associated with minimizing reports of use. However, no published study has examined how social desirability affects self-reports of social network variables among substance abusers. If it is found, for example, that socially desirable responding affects reports of others' substance use or support for use from others, then it may be important for future researchers and clinicians to control for these tendencies when having individuals report on the socially undesirable behaviors of others.

In the present study, the relationship between the two aspects of social desirability and self-reports of social support variables on Clifford and colleagues' (Clifford & Longabaugh, 1991; Clifford, Longabaugh, & Beattie, 1992) Important People Inventory were examined within a group recovery home sample. Given that substance abusers tend to falsely report substance abuse, it was expected that recovering substance abusers living in Oxford House group recovery homes would unrealistically inflate reports of social support (i.e., higher general support, fewer drinking behaviors of friends and family, and less support for drinking from social contacts). It also was hypothesized that lower self-deception scores would predict more positive social support variables over time. If persons in recovery become more "honest" with themselves, then their support systems may improve.

METHOD

Participants

Participants were 582 adults (67.7% men, 32.3% women; M age = 39.6 years old, SD = 9.3) who completed the Balanced Inventory of Desirable Responding at two data collection waves (i.e., Waves 2 and 4). This sample was drawn from a larger 2-year U.S. nationwide longitudinal study (see Jason, Davis, Ferrari, & Anderson, 2007) containing 897 Oxford House group home residents at the start of the study. Founded in 1975, Oxford House (OH) provides a national network of supportive, democratic, self-run, communal-living settings for recovering substance abusers. Because residents maintain financial responsibility by paying for their own rent, food, and utilities, and by sharing in house chores, OH is no more expensive than any other place of residence. Residents may stay indefinitely, provided that they pay rent, abstain from alcohol and drug use, and avoid disruptive behavior. Additionally, OH is completely devoid of professional therapists or treatment providers (Ferrari, Jason, Olson, Davis, & Alvarez, 2002; Jason, Ferrari, Dvorchak, Groessl, & Malloy, 1997).

The sample was ethnically diverse, with 57.8% European American, 34.6% African American, 3.4% Hispanic/Latino, and 4.3% others. At the start of the study, the average education level was 12.7 years (SD = 2.0). With respect to employment, 71.3% reported being employed full-time, 13.3% worked part-time, 10.9% were unemployed, and 4.5% were retired or disabled. The average monthly income of participants was $1014.70 ($SD$ = 850.6). In the 90 days previous to entry into the study, 9.6% of participants reported using alcohol, and 7.3% reported using illicit drugs. On average, participants had undergone alcohol treatment of 2.6 times (SD = 3.6) and drug treatment 2.9 times (SD = 3.3) during their lives. The average length of abstinence from alcohol was 2.1 years (SD = 3.0) and 2.2 years (SD = 3.3) for drugs.

Procedure

The majority of participants were recruited through an announcement published in a monthly newsletter circulated throughout these recovery home settings. Members of the research team then contacted the homes via letters to house presidents, conducted follow-up phone calls to the houses, and where possible, arranged to visit the houses. The remainder of participants were recruited at an annual Oxford House convention. Analyses of data collected at the convention versus data collected using the first method did not reveal significant differences in outcome or sociodemographic variables. This study was approved by an institutional review board; thus, all attempts were made to adhere to ethical standards. The nature, purpose, and goals of the study were explained to potential participants. Informed consent was given, and research team members explained that participation was entirely voluntary and withdrawal from the study was possible at any time. Furthermore, participants were assured that their responses would remain confidential. Payments of $15 were made to participants following each survey. We focused on two measurement waves (i.e., Waves 2 and 4) from the Jason et al. (2007) data set separated by an 8-month period. Correlations were run between the 11 *IP* indices and the two social desirability constructs (i.e., self-deception and impression management). Additionally, linear regression analyses were run to determine if Wave 2 self-deception scores predicted social support variables at Wave 4.

Measures

At both data collection waves, participants completed the Important People Inventory (IP, Clifford & Longabaugh, 1991; Clifford et al., 1992). This structured interview required participants to identify important members in their networks with whom they frequently contacted within the past 6 months. In the first section of the IP, labeled the Important People section, a participant was asked to identify up to 12 social contacts over the age of 12 years. For each person the participant listed in his or her network, the inventory examined the type of relationship, the duration of relationship in years, and the frequency of contact. In addition, the participant assessed how often the network member drank, how much the network member drank on a maximum drinking day, and the network member's overall drinking status. In the next section, called the Most Important People (MIP) section, the participant chose up to four network members who were the most important over the past 6 months. The participant then rated each network member's importance, how much he or she liked the person, and how the person reacted to the participant's drinking. The current study utilized the nine-index, three-factor model of the IP proposed by Groh, Olson, Jason, Ferrari, and Davis (2007), namely: (a) General Social Support (indices 1–3; initial wave Cronbach's alpha = 0.33); (b) Drinking Behaviors of Network Members (indices 4,7,8; initial wave Cronbach's alpha = 0.78); and, (c) Support for Drinking from Network Members (indices 9–11; initial wave Cronbach's alpha = 0.81). This model has good internal reliability and is structurally supported by factor analyses. Individual mean scores are not interpretable due to standardization of the 11 indices before computing the factor scores.

Several researchers customized the IP to assess support specific to participants' illicit drug use in addition to alcohol use (see Jason, Olson, Ferrari, & Lo Sasso, 2006; Jason et al., 2007; Majer, Jason, Ferrari, Venable, & Olson, 2002; Schmitt, 2003). Because it is possible that social support for drug use has an even greater association with self-deception because of the stigmatized nature of drug as opposed to alcohol use, we focused on support for drug use in addition to alcohol use in the present study. To assess drug use, a few additional questions were added. The questions that contributed to the alcohol-specific indices (i.e., indices 4, 7–11) were repeated, but with the words "drinking" altered to "drug use." Likewise, the alcohol-related composite scores were accordingly changed.

In addition, participants completed Paulhus's (1998) Balanced Inventory of Desirable Responding (BIDR). This scale contained 40 items rated along a 7-point Likert-type response scale (1 = *not true*; 7 = *very true*). Unlike other similar measures (e.g., the Marlowe-Crowne Social Desirability Scale [Crowne & Marlow, 1960]), the BIDR separated social desirability into two separate but related concepts, each measured by 20-items: self-enhancement and impression management. The self-deceptive enhancement subscale ($M = 81.10$, $SD = 12.91$), which examined a person's tendency to engage in statements that enhance or exaggerate one's abilities and skills, was administered at Wave 2 of the larger study. In contrast, the impression management subscale ($M = 81.93$, $SD = 18.78$), an assessment of one's self-presentation style to favorably impress others, was administered at Wave 4, 8 months later. Paulhus (1988) reported Cronbach's alphas between 0.74 and 0.86 for the two subscales, respectively, and the alphas in the present study were 0.65 and 0.78, respectively. Factor analyses of the scale conducted by the scale's author demonstrated strong discriminant validity for both subscales across numerous other response distortion scales (see Paulhus, 1984, 1988; Paulhus & Reid, 1991). Paulhus (1994) authorized two scoring methods of the BIDR: continuous (i.e., all answers are utilized) and dichotomous (i.e., only extreme scores are utilized). Because the continuous scoring method has demonstrated stronger convergent and internal validity (see Stober, Dette, & Musch, 2002), we decided in the present study to use the continuous scoring method in all data analyses.

RESULTS

Regarding social support networks, of a possible 12 people, participants listed an average of 6.5 ($SD = 3.5$) members in their social networks.

Regarding gender, 52.2% of network members were male, and 47.8% were female. The mean length of relationship was 14.3 ($SD = 9.7$) years, and participants on average had contact with members about once or twice a week. Almost all network members were considered to be generally supportive (98.0%). About three quarters (74.8%) of network members abstained from alcohol or were in alcohol recovery; 91.1% of network contacts abstained from illegal drugs or were in drug abuse recovery.

For all outcome analyses, the probability level was set at .01 in order to control for Type 1 error. To test the relationship between self-deception and self-reported general and alcohol-specific social support variables, correlations were run between the 11 IP indices and BIDR self-deception scores at Wave 2 (see Table 1). Results indicated that self-deception scores were significantly related to number of people in the network, $r(535) = -.12$,

TABLE 1 Zero-order Correlates between Social Desirability and IP Scores

Index Number/Composite Score	Self-deception	Impression Management
1. Number of people in the network	−.12*	.08
2. Amount of contact with one's network	.08	.04
3. Average importance of most important people	.08	.03
4a. Drinking status of network members	−.09	−.07
4d. Drug use status of network members	−.07	−.04
5a. Frequency with which network members drink	−.08	−.09
5d. Frequency with which network members use drugs	.01	−.04
6a. Maximum drinking of network members on a drinking day	−.03	−.06
6d. Maximum drug use of network members on a drug using day	−.02	−.02
7a. Percentage of heavy drinkers in the network	−.06	−.12*
7d. Percentage of heavy drug users in the network	−.08	−.13*
8a. Percentage of abstainers and recovering alcoholics in the network	.01	.17**
8d. Percentage of abstainers and recovering drug addicts in the network	.06	.18**
9a. Most support for drinking among most important people	−.05	−.07
9d. Most support for drug use among most important people	−.00	−.04
10a. Least support for drinking among most important people	.07	−.07
10d. Least support for drug use among most important people	.09	−.03
11a. Average support for drinking among most important people	.04	−.02
11d. Average support for drug use among most important people	.08	−.02
General Social Support Composite Score	.02	.07
Drinking Behaviors of Network Members Composite Score	−.06	−.15*
Drug Use Behaviors of Network Members Composite Score	−.08	−.13*
Support for Drinking from Network Members Composite Score	.03	−.06
Support for Drug Use from Network Members Composite Score	.07	−.03

Note, a = alcohol use index, d = drug use index. *$p < .01$. **$p < .001$.

$p = .007$. Individuals with high self-deceptive tendencies were more likely to report having social support networks that were smaller. These self-deception analyses were run again, with the focus on support for drug use instead of alcohol use for the relevant indices (i.e., 4 through 11), but significant relationships were not found.

Next we correlated the 11 IP indices with scores for the second BIDR subscale, impression management, at Wave 4 (see Table 1). Results indicated that impression management scores were significantly related to percentage of heavy drinkers in the network, $r(527) = -.12$, $p = .005$, and percentage of abstainers and recovering alcoholics in the network, $r(527) = .17$, $p = .000$. In other words, individuals with high impression management tendencies were more likely to report having social support networks containing a lower percentage of heavy drinkers and a lower percentage of abstainers and recovering drug addicts. In addition, the Drinking Behaviors of Network Members composite score had a significant relationship with impression management, $r(527) = -.15$, $p = .001$. Individuals with high impression management were more likely to report that their network contacts displayed fewer drinking behaviors. Concerning drug use, self-deception had a significant positive relationship with percentage of heavy drug users in the network, $r(581) = .13$, $p = .003$, and a significant negative relationship with percentage of abstainers and recovering drug addicts in the network, $r(526) = .18$, $p = .000$. In addition, the Drug Use Behaviors of Network Members composite score was found to have a significant negative relationship with self-deception, $r(582) = -.13$, $p = .002$.

Because the impression management subscale was only given at Wave 4, we were unable to longitudinally examine the influence of this construct. However, since the IP was administered at all waves, and the self-deception subscale of the BIDR was administered at Wave 2, we were able to test longitudinally the influence of self-deception on social support over an 8-month time period. Specifically, linear regression analyses were run to determine if Wave 2 self-deception scores predicted social support variables at Wave 4 (see Table 2). Five separate models were run: self-deception was the predictor variable in each case, and the outcome variables included the different IP composite scores. The only statistically significant regression model included self-deception, predicting lower Drinking Behaviors of Network Members scores, $\beta = -.12$, $t(525) = -2.68$, $p = .007$. Thus, individuals with greater tendencies toward self-deception at Wave 2 reported having fewer friends and family members who consumed alcohol at Wave 4. As suggested earlier in this article, it is believed that participants with these socially desirability biases misrepresented their social support networks to appear more favorable to others. However, it is important to note that the effect sizes for these significant relations were low.

TABLE 2 Summary of Regression Analyses for Self-Deception Scores Predicting Social Support Variables

Model	B	$SE\ B$	β
1. Self-deception predicting *General social support*	.01	.13	.003
2. Self-deception predicting *Drinking behaviors of network members*	−.44	.16	−.12*
3. Self-deception predicting *Drug use behaviors of network members*	−.17	.17	−.04
4. Self-deception predicting *Support for drinking from network members*	−.02	.18	−.01
5. Self-deception predicting *Support for drug use from network members*	.14	.18	.04

$n = 526$, *$p < .01$.

DISCUSSION

Data from correlational and regression analyses suggest that participants residing in communal-living recovery homes (i.e., Oxford Houses) might have reported certain social network variables in a socially desirable manner (although effect sizes were low). Notably, most of the significant relations with social desirability variables focused on the drinking and drug use habits of important network contacts. Perhaps the reporting of friends and family members' substance use within a communal-living recovery sample was a more sensitive issue than the reporting of general support or support for drinking. This pattern is consistent with other research emphasizing friendships with abstainers and decreasing friendships with users common to various treatments ranging from cognitive-behavioral therapy (e.g., Bandura, 1986) to 12-step and mutual-help models (Humphreys & Noke, 1997). It may be difficult for communal-living residents (many of whom also attend 12-step programs) to report that their important social contacts are using drugs and alcohol when they receive so much pressure to avoid spending time with these individuals. Because of this finding, future researchers may choose to control for these tendencies when having individuals report on the socially undesirable behaviors of their friends and family.

A surprising finding was that more significant relations with social desirability were seen for alcohol-specific social support than drug-specific social support variables. This may suggest that alcohol-related social support in this sample was more prone to social desirability than drug-related support. We originally expected that social support for drug use would have a greater association with self-deception due to the greater stigma associated with illicit drug use. However, this reversed effect might have been found because more participants used alcohol than drugs in the past 3 months (suggesting more recent alcohol use in this sample); thus, participants would have more reason to misrepresent alcohol than drug use.

There were several limitations in the present study. To start out with, the results were mostly correlational in nature; thus, causal relations cannot be assumed. Overall, effect sizes were low, so alternate explanations are certainly possible besides the effects of social desirability; however, the probability level was set at .01 in order to control for Type 1 error. In addition, the General Social Support composite score of the IP had low internal reliability, which may help explain the general lack of significant findings for this factor. Also, it was not possible to compare the results for impression management and self-deception subscales because these measures were administered one year apart. The inability to show that time 1 self-deception predicted reports of substance use by others at time 2 while controlling for time 2 self-deception scores provides another weakness of this study.

Furthermore, some selection bias might have occurred, and the low rates of current alcohol and drug use by participants may indicate that only the more successful or motivated Oxford House residents participated and completed the necessary measures. Perhaps, future research assessing self-deception should consider a sample with more variability with regards to substance use and stages of recovery. It has also been argued that Oxford House residents represent a self-selected sample within the substance abuse recovery population. Research by Jason, Davis, Ferrari, and Bishop (2001) refuted this claim, however, demonstrating that the demographic profile of Oxford House residents matches the typical profile of recovering alcoholics in traditional treatment settings. Even so, findings might not generalize to others in recovery for several reasons. First of all, because Oxford House residents as a rule reside with friends instead of family, perhaps social support is very different in these settings. For example, support provided by friends is likely more essential for this sample than for others in recovery, for whom support from family is more essential. Additionally, OH residents must be sober upon entry into the program and may be further along in their recovery than people in other treatments. Consequently, it cannot be said that social support and social desirability play the exact same role in recovery for those who are not yet at that stage. In addition, OH provides a highly structured abstinent environment, and perhaps social support and social desirability play a different role in the real world, which contains less structure and more opportunities for substance use and criminal behavior.

In any case, social desirability is a major concern when working with substance abuse populations, and it is important to attempt to understand these types of biases. The present study indicated that similar to self-reports of substance use, self-reports of social network variables might also susceptible to social desirable responding (particularly in structured residential recovery settings such as Oxford House). BIDR social desirability scores demonstrated relationships with several social network characteristics, in particular those focusing on the drinking behaviors of one's friends and family. Therefore, it may be important for clinicians and researchers to assess self-deception and impression management when utilizing self-reports of social networks or other potentially socially undesirable variables within substance abuse populations.

REFERENCES

Bandura, A. (1986). *Social foundations of thought and action: A social cognitive theory.* Englewood Cliffs, NJ: Prentice-Hall.

Bradburn, N. (1983). Response effects. In P. Rossi, J. Wright, & A. Anderson (Eds.), *Handbook of survey research.* New York: Academic Press.

Clifford, P. R., & Longabaugh, R. (1991). *Manual for the administration of the Important People and Activities instrument: Adapted for use by Project MATCH.* Unpublished document. Center for Alcohol and Addiction Studies, Brown University: Providence, RI.

Clifford, P. R., Longabaugh, R., & Beattie, M. (1992). Social support and patient drinking: A validation study (Abstract). *Alcoholism: Clinical and Experimental Research, 16,* 403.

Cohen, S., Underwood, L. G., & Gottlieb, B. H. (2000). *Social support measurement and intervention.* New York: Oxford University Press.

Cohen, S., & Wills, T. A. (1985). Stress, social support, and the buffering hypothesis. *Psychological Bulletin, 98,* 310–357.

Cox, B. J., Swinson, R. P., Direnfield, D. M., & Bourdeau, D. (1994). Social desirability and self-reports of alcohol-abuse in anxiety disorder patients. *Behaviour Research and Therapy, 32,* 175–178.

Crowne, D. P., & Marlowe, D. (1960). A new scale of social desirability independent of psychopathology. *Journal of Consulting Psychology, 24,* 349–354.

Falkin, G. P., & Strauss, S. M. (2003). Social supporters and drug use enablers: A dilemma for women in recovery. *Addictive Behaviors, 28,* 141–155.

Ferrari, J. R., Jason, L. A., Olson, B. D., Davis, M. I., & Alvarez, J. (2002). Sense of community among Oxford House residents recovering from substance abuse: Making a house a home. In. A. T. Fischer, C. C. Sonn, & B. J. Bishop (Eds.), *Psychological sense of community* (pp. 109–122). New York: Kluwer/Plenum.

Finney, J., Moos, R., & Mewborn, R. (1980). Posttreatment experiences and treatment outcome of alcoholic patients six months and two years after hospitalization. *Journal of Consulting and Clinical Psychology, 48,* 17–29.

Groh, D. R., Olson, B. D., Jason, L. A., Ferrari, J. R., & Davis, M. I. (2007). A factor analysis of the Important People Inventory. *Alcohol & Alcoholism, 42,* 347–353.

Haber, M. G., Cohen, J. L., Lucas, T., & Baltes, B. B. (2007). The relationship between self-reported received and perceived social support: A meta-analytic review. *American Journal of Community Psychology, 39,* 133–144.

Humphreys, K., & Noke, J. M. (1997). The influence of posttreatment mutual help group participation on the friendship networks of substance abuse patients. *American Journal of Community Psychology, 25,* 1–16.

Jason, L. A., Davis, M. I., Ferrari, J. R., & Anderson, E. (2007). The need for substance abuse after-care: A longitudinal analysis of Oxford House. *Addictive Behaviors, 32*, 803–818.

Jason, L. A., Davis, M. I., Ferrari, J. R., & Bishop, P. D. (2001). Oxford House: A review of research and implications for substance abuse recovery and community research. *Journal of Drug Education, 31*, 1–27.

Jason, L. A., Ferrari, J. R., Dvorchak, P. A., Groessl, E. J., & Malloy, J. P. (1997). The characteristics of alcoholics in self-help residential treatment settings: A multi-site study of Oxford House. *Alcoholism Treatment Quarterly, 15*, 53–63.

Jason, L. A., Olson, B. D., Ferrari, J. R., & Lo Sasso, A. T. (2006). Communal housing settings enhance substance abuse recovery. *American Journal of Public Health, 91*, 1727–1729.

Longabaugh, R., & Beattie, M. C. (1986). Social investment, environmental support and treatment outcomes of alcoholics. *Alcohol Health and Research World, Summer*, 64–66.

Majer, J. M., Jason, L. A., Ferrari, J. R., Venable, L. B., & Olson, B. D. (2002). Social support and self-efficacy for abstinence: Is peer identification an issue? *Journal of Substance Abuse Treatment, 23*, 209–215.

Paulhus, D. L. (1984). Two-component models of socially desirable responding. *Journal of Personality & Social Psychology, 46*, 598–609.

Paulhus, D. L. (1988). Measurement and control of response bias. In J. P. Robinson, P. Shaver, & L. Wrightsman (Eds.), *Measures of personality and social psychological attitudes* (Vol. 1, pp. 17–60). New York: Academic Press.

Paulhus, D. L. (1991). Measurement and control of response bias. In J. P. Robinson, P. R. Shaver, & L. S. Wrightsman (Eds.), *Measures of personality and social psychological attitudes* (pp. 17–59). San Diego, CA: Academic Press.

Paulhus, D. L. (1994). *Balanced Inventory of Desirable Responding: Reference manual for BIDR version 6*. Unpublished manuscript. Department of Psychology, University of British Colombia, Vancouver, Canada.

Paulhus, D. L. (1998). *Manual for the balanced inventory of desirable responding (BIDR-7)*. Toronto, Ontario, Canada: Multi-Health Systems.

Paulhus, D. L., & Reid, D. B. (1991). Enhancement and denial in socially desirable responding. *Journal of Personality and Social Psychology, 60*, 307–371.

Richards, H. J., & Pai, S. M. (2003). Deception in prison assessment of substance abuse. *Journal of Substance Abuse Treatment, 24*, 121–128.

Rychtarik, R. G., Tarnowski, K. T., & St. Lawrence, J. S. (1989). Impact of social desirability response sets on the self-report of marital adjustment in alcoholics. *Journal of Studies on Alcohol, 50*, 1989.

Schmitt, M. M. (2003). Recovery from substance abuse: The role of unsupportive social interactions. *Dissertation Abstracts International, 64 (2-B)*, 974.

Stober, J., Dette, D. E., & Musch, J. (2002). Comparing continuous and dichotomous scoring of the balanced inventory of desirable responding. *Journal of Personality Assessment, 78*, 370–389.

Sense of Community within Oxford House Recovery Housing: Impact of Resident Age and Income

BENJAMIN C. GRAHAM, MS, LEONARD A. JASON, PhD, and
JOSEPH R. FERRARI, PhD

DePaul University

MARGARET I. DAVIS, PhD

Dickinson College

The experience of psychological sense of community (PSOC) can play an important role in the substance abuse recovery process. This study explored the relationship between PSOC and setting-level variables of age and income among residents living in Oxford House, a communal, self-governed recovery housing model (n = 70). Age and income variables were not related to an overall PSOC or components such as shared common mission or feelings of reciprocal responsibility. However, both age and income variables were significant predictors of the harmony felt within these houses. The role that PSOC may play in recovery facilities and other co-housing arrangements was discussed, and implications for future research and application were outlined.

If a person described the significant nonfamily relationships within their life, the ensuing narrative would likely include what community psychologists call a *psychological sense of community* (*PSOC*: Sarason, 1974). This construct refers to the sense of belongingness that members feel within a group possessing shared values and emotional connection (McMillan & Chavis, 1986). In addition, these communities possess the capacity to influence and be influenced by their members (McMillan & Chavis, 1986). Over the past 3 decades, community psychology has generated a body of research on the experience of PSOC (see Fisher, Sonn, & Bishop, 2002). When facing a significant behavioral change, such as remaining abstinent from drugs and alcohol, it is possible that individuals rely on social supports experienced from a positive PSOC (Ferrari, Jason, Davis, Olson, & Alvarez, 2004).

More recently, definitions of PSOC stressed the contextual nature of the construct. Since Sarason's (1974) acknowledgement that PSOC varies by situation and over time, many studies explored specific contextual and cultural definitions of PSOC (Bishop, Colquhoun, & Johnson, 2006; Hill, 1996). Another trend in the theory of PSOC focused on multiple levels of analysis, on both the individual and group level (Hill, 1996). Finally, contemporary research on PSOC explored how the construct of PSOC related to other similar constructs, such as group cohesion, social support, acculturation, and collective efficacy (Proescholdbell & Roosa, 2005).

Few studies examined PSOC within substance abuse recovery settings, such as Oxford House—a self-run, democratic, mutual aid co-housing movement for persons in recovery (Oxford House, Inc., n.d.). Founded in 1975, the Oxford House model facilitates an environment where persons in recovery live together, managing their household as a collective unit. Oxford House households average eight same-sex residents and operate with a universal rule that participants stay totally sober. Rules also extend to day-to-day tasks such as routine chores and behavior related to conflict management. The primary decision-making forum is a weekly house meeting in which an 80% majority vote is needed for house decisions (Ferrari et al., 2004; Oxford House, Inc., n.d.). Currently, over 1,200 Oxford Houses exist in the United States, Australia, and Canada.

Social support for abstinence is a tenet of Oxford House. Each Oxford House is open to anyone committed to staying sober, regardless of her or his background. This value of diversity is expressed in the culturally diverse groups of individuals who live within Oxford Houses, including a significant number of houses for women and women with children. Furthermore, the individual members within each house vary among individual characteristics such as age, income, type of employment, and educational level (see Jason, Ferrari, Dvorchak, Groessl, & Malloy, 1997). Up to this point, only a limited number of studies have explored how such heterogeneity of residents impacts the psychological experience of Oxford House residents.

Several studies explored house characteristics in the Oxford House experience (e.g., Ferrari, Jason, Sasser, Davis, & Olson, 2006; Ferrari et al., 2004; Jason, Ferrari, Freeland, Danielewicz, & Olson, 2005). One study found that Oxford Houses, compared to traditional therapeutic communities, were more likely to set rules around destructive setting-level behaviors (e.g., vandalism), extend greater personal liberties to members, and allow personal possessions to be brought into the house (Ferrari et al., 2004). In another study that examined house business meetings, it was found that these meetings functioned largely as a forum to address procedural and day-to-day issues at the house level, rather than an opportunity to delve into matters pertaining to specific residents (Jason et al., 2005). Finally, Ferrari et al. (2006) found Oxford Houses to possess well-maintained interior and exterior characteristics, suggesting that setting-level factors may create a greater sense of home.

In general, PSOC is strengthened the longer a person is part of a community (Hill, 1996; Skjaeveland, Garling, & Maeland, 1996). Research on Oxford House participants indicated that a primary reason individuals chose to become members was the camaraderie and abstinence social support they received within the setting (Jason, Ferrari, Smith, Marsh, Dvorchak, & Groessl, 1997; Ferrari, Jason, Olson, Davis, & Alvarez, 2002). Although both female and male residents reported valuing social support in recovery, women placed greater emphasis on social supports than did men (Kim, Davis, Jason, & Ferrari, 2006). This sense of fellowship among residents increased the longer members stayed in an Oxford House (Bishop, Jason, Ferrari, & Huang, 1998).

Bishop et al. (1997) surveyed males living in Oxford House and found that the difference in an individual's age and the cohort age of his Oxford House was a significant predictor for how long the individual chose to stay in the house. Results indicated that persons with larger differences in age from the average house age reported staying *longer* in the house. It was suggested that in recovery communities, younger members may benefit from the experiential knowledge of older members, and the oldest members benefit from the helper principle. Thus, age outliers of a house were more likely to stay for longer periods (Bishop et al., 1997).

In addition to age, it is likely that income, and the range of income within houses, is related to PSOC. As described above, Oxford House is a self-run model that emphasizes a house's financial self-sustainability as well as solidarity among members around sobriety. Income relates to these guiding principles such that the composite of each individual's income affects the stability of these rented dwellings. Furthermore, the value that each Oxford House places on abstinence asserts that this shared connection may be more powerful than the similarity of members' socioeconomic status.

The findings of Bishop et al. (1997) on age, as well as the hypothesis that income diversity is positive for the PSOC of a house, exist within a broader body of research on groups, where there is not a clear consensus on the role of heterogeneity or homogeneity in predicting group experience. Work groups have been examined in regard to performance on different types of tasks, and it was found that tasks requiring creative judgment making benefited from group heterogeneity (McGrath, 1984), while demographic homogeneity was found to result in greater group cohesiveness (Jackson, 1992). The general research on age diversity within groups suggests that groups with wider age diversity had higher turnover rates and lower reported group cohesion (Jackson, 1992). For example, attitudes and values have been shown to vary as a function of age cohort (Elder, 1975; Oakes, 2003).

There is a clear need to better understand the role that demographic heterogeneity or homogeneity plays in Oxford House settings, including psychological constructs such as PSOC. Ferrari et al. (2002) have described the PSOC that members experience as a critical component to the success of the Oxford House model and have called for further research to better understand how PSOC contributes to and is influenced by other factors in the Oxford House experience. One area that has only begun to be explored in Oxford House is the extent to which the interpersonal dynamics of a household have on an individual's experience of his or her house. Given that social support is reported as one of the driving motivations for persons entering Oxford House, advancing knowledge regarding correlates of PSOC is warranted (Jason, Ferrari, Smith, et al., 1997).

The present study addresses this need by exploring how characteristics of age and income among persons living in Oxford Houses related to overall household PSOC. By pooling PSOC scores for a specific house, the present study explored how resident characteristics of age and income related to overall house PSOC. This study contributes to the growing consensus that PSOC research should utilize multiple levels of analysis, not simply individual-level exploration (see Brodsky, O'Campo, & Aronson, 1999; Hill, 1996). Furthermore, our understanding of PSOC within Oxford Houses would expand the "extraindividual"-level construct of community (Proescholdbell & Roosa, 2005) from the individual to group level. In addition, the present study outlined a method for creating house-level variables from individual data. We expected houses with high age heterogeneity to report a higher PSOC than houses with low age heterogeneity. Also, houses with high-income heterogeneity were expected to report a higher PSOC than houses with low-income heterogeneity.

METHOD

This study was a secondary data analysis using data described from the study of Jason, Ferrari, Dvorchak, Groessl, and Malloy (1997) consisting of 897 individuals living in 214 different Oxford Houses in the United States. For each of the 214 houses, the number of participants per household ranged from a single individual to every member of the house. Therefore, it was necessary to establish a method of filtering households with low representation to preserve the robustness of our house-level variables. A dummy variable with a ratio score between 0 and 1 was constructed to explore house-level data. The ratio was calculated by dividing the number of individuals participating in the study by the total number of beds in that specific house. This coefficient reflected the percentage of members representing the individual house.

In order to merge individual-level variables into house-level variables, we sought houses with a relatively high member representation. A house ratio score of 0.70 (i.e., 70% member representation) was set as the cutoff ratio score for a house to be included in the present study. This cutoff reduced the sample to 70 houses from the original 214.

All Oxford Houses are same sex in composition. Of the 70 houses, 66% settings were male and 34% were female, and residents reported a mean age of 38 years ($SD = 5.17$). The mean income across houses from all sources of revenue in a given month was \$802.42 ($SD = 398.20). Houses were coded as having heterogeneous race or ethnicity membership, homogenous European American membership, or homogenous African American membership, yielding 81.4% ($n = 57$) of settings in the present sample as heterogeneous. A minority of houses were ethnically or racially homogenous, with 11.4% ($n = 8$) of these houses being European American and 7.1% ($n = 5$) African American. It should be noted that there were significant Latino/Hispanic non-White, Native American, and other representations within houses such that no house setting consisted exclusively of members from any of these ethnic or racial groups.

The primary data consisted of PSOC scale scores, monthly income, and chronological age. The PSOC scale used was Bishop, Chertok, and Jason's (1997) 30-item, 5-point Likert (1 = *not at all true*, 5 = *completely true*) *perceived sense of community scale*. Scores on this scale were divided into three subscales, namely, (a) *mission* (12 items: "There is a sense of common purpose in this group"), referring to the sense of mission that members feel in the group's purpose, (b) *reciprocal responsibility* (12 items: "There is a feeling that the group looks out for its members"), the belief that members help one another in a reciprocal way, and (c) *harmony* (6 items: "There are definite "in" and "out" groups within this group"), whether or not members perceived harmony existing within the group. The individual PSOC scores for each house were averaged, creating a single house-level variable for each PSOC score. Standard deviations of age and income were calculated for each house based on individual data.

RESULTS

Gender, geographic location, and race or ethnicity of houses were controlled for in initial stages of analysis. The geographic location variable comprised of four different regions in the United States. House gender, geographic location, and race or ethnicity were not found to be significant predictors of PSOC. Separate regressions then were run for the four scores associated with the PSOC scores (i.e., total score, harmony subscale, mission subscale, and reciprocity subscale). The model consisted of house age heterogeneity and house income heterogeneity as independent variables. House age

TABLE 1 Summary of Regression Analysis for Variables Predicting PSOC-Harmony Scores

Variable	B	SE B	β
Age heterogeneity	.0413	.017	.275*
Income heterogeneity	.0003	.000	.283*

($n = 70$ facilities).
*p < .05.

heterogeneity consisted of the standard deviation of member ages within a given house. Similarly, house income heterogeneity was measured by the standard deviation of monthly incomes of a house's members. Of the four analyses, the only significant model included harmony subscale scores. Both age and income were significant predictors for levels of harmony across houses, $F (2,67) = 5.86$, $p < .01$ (see Table 1). The greater the heterogeneity for both age and income, the higher reported levels of reported house harmony.

DISCUSSION

The Oxford House model of recovery states that the common bond of staying sober unites house members regardless of how dissimilar they are as individuals (Oxford House, Inc., n.d.). The present study found some support for this hypothesis, in that houses with wider age and income ranges reported a higher level of harmony. This finding was consistent with some of the previous research on Oxford House (Ferrari et al., 2002), as well as research on task performance involving creativity suggesting that groups have better outcomes when a diversity of perspectives exists (Jackson, 1992). However, the results of the present study contrast with other research that suggests likeness as an asset to group identity (Byrne, 1971). Results offer support for the notion that diverse groups can experience a high sense of harmony when united around a common purpose.

Previous research on Oxford House identified a mentoring relationship that took place between older and younger residents, such that members on the extremes of the house age range were more likely to stay in the house for a longer period of time (Bishop et al., 1997, 1998). The group-level variable of age heterogeneity employed in this study provided further support for this claim, in that houses with larger age heterogeneity reported a higher sense of harmony. In addition, the finding that larger income heterogeneity was related to a higher harmony score is noteworthy. A possible interpretation is that the presence of one or two high-earning individuals in the house positively influenced the sense of harmony members felt in the house. It has been postulated that the presence of members who were established financially and professionally provided positive role modeling for other members trying to readjust in society after years of addiction (P. Malloy, personal communication, 2006).

One policy implication of this study is the affirmation that the formation of future Oxford Houses, and potentially other co-housing recovery settings, should not be constricted to demographically similar residents (specifically in regard to age and income). Moreover, identifying potential residents across a wide range of age and income may actually strengthen the ability of the home environment to promote recovery. It is important to note that, of the three PSOC subscale scores (mission, reciprocal responsibility, harmony) only harmony scores were significantly related to age and income heterogeneity. The lack of correlation of relationship between age or income heterogeneity to mission scores was consistent with the Oxford House notion of solidarity across age and income. Nevertheless, the null finding of reciprocal responsibility should be interpreted with caution. On the one hand, reciprocal responsibility should (like mission), be equal regardless of the level of house age or income heterogeneity. It is likely that mentor-mentee relationships existed across age and income ranges within houses (i.e., older and more established residents providing unreciprocated support to younger and less financially stable residents). Due to the complexities of the various types of reciprocal supports occurring at any given house, it may be that the 12 items that comprised the reciprocal responsibility subscale lacked the specificity to fully examine the phenomena.

Co-housing structures offer an efficient, supportive and economical way of living for various groups as they work toward their common goals. Oxford House is one model that demonstrates the potential benefits of this type of group structure. Other populations might benefit from similar models (e.g., persons with chronic mental illness, persons with chronic physical illness and dual diagnosis populations, as well as single parent families). Historically, informal forms of mutual aid among these groups existed (e.g., single-parent families sharing resources for childcare or housing, cancer survivors' groups), but a more developed model of co-housing was not available. In other cases models do exist, such as co-housing for elderly persons, but have been implemented in only a limited capacity (Prosper, Sherman, & Howe, 2004). Findings from this study suggest that policies that promote such housing arrangements should not assume that likeness indicates a more cohesive group environment. Diverse perspectives on a shared experience may in fact increase the level of group connection in supportive group settings.

The construct of PSOC is a useful tool in understanding co-housing operations. A major success of the Oxford House model may be attributed to the positive psychological sense of community experienced by residents. The present study provided support for the shared experience of living together under a common vision superseding individual differences among communal-living residents. Further PSOC research on co-housing has the potential to assist not only persons in recovery, but other co-housing populations organized around a shared purpose.

REFERENCES

Bishop, B., Colquhoun, S., & Johnson, G. (2006). Psychological sense of community: An Australian Aboriginal experience. *Journal of Community Psychology, 34*, 1–7.

Bishop, P. D., Chertok, F., & Jason, L. A. (1997). Measuring sense of community: Beyond local boundaries. *Journal of Primary Prevention, 18*, 193–212.

Bishop, P. D., Jason, L. A., Ferrari, J. R., & Huang, C. F. (1998). A survival analysis of communal-living, self-help, addiction recovery participants. *American Journal of Community Psychology, 26*, 803–821.

Brodsky, A. E., O'Campo, P. J., & Aronson, R. E. (1999). PSOC in community context: Multi-level correlates of a measure of psychological sense of community in low-income, urban neighborhoods. *Journal of Community Psychology, 27*, 659–679.

Byrne, D. (1971). *The attraction paradigm*. New York: Academic Press.

Elder, G. H. (1975). Age differentiation and the life course. *Annual Review of Sociology, 1*, 165–190.

Ferrari, J. R., Jason, L. A., Davis, M. I., Olson, B. D., & Alvarez, J. (2004). Similarities and differences in governance among residents in drug and/or alcohol misuse and recovery: Self vs. staff rules and regulations. *Therapeutic Communities, 25*, 185–198.

Ferrari, J. R., Jason, L. A., Olson, B. D., Davis, M. I., & Alvarez, J. (2002). Sense of community among Oxford House residents recovering from substance abuse: Making a house a home. In A. T. Fischer, C. C. Sonn, & B. J. Bishop (Eds.), *Psychological sense of community: Research, applications and implications* (pp. 109–122). New York: Kluwer/Plenum.

Ferrari, J. R., Jason, L. A., Sasser, K. C., Davis, M. I., & Olson, B. I. (2006). Creating a home to promote recovery: The physical environments of Oxford House. *Journal of Prevention & Intervention in the Community, 31*, 27–40.

Fisher, A. T., Sonn, C. C., & Bishop, B. J. (Eds.). (2002). *Psychological sense of community: Research, applications, and implications*. New York: Kluwer/Plenum.

Hill, J. L. (1996). Psychological sense of community: Suggestions for future research. *Journal of Community Psychology, 24*, 431–438.

Jackson, S. E. (1992). Team composition in organizational settings: Issues in managing an increasingly diverse work force. In S. Worchel, W. Wood, & J. A. Simpson (Eds.), *Group process and productivity* (pp. 138–173). Newbury Park, CA: Sage.

Jason, L. A., Ferrari J. R., Dvorchak, P. A., Groessl, E. J., & Malloy, P. J. (1997). The characteristics of alcoholics in self-help residential treatment settings: A multi-site study of Oxford House. *Alcoholism Treatment Quarterly, 15*, 53–63.

Jason, L. A., Ferrari, J. R., Freeland, M., Danielewicz, J., & Olson, B. (2005). Observing organizational and interaction behaviors among mutual-help recovery home members. *International Journal of Self Help and Self Care, 3*, 117–132.

Jason, L. A., Ferrari J. R., Smith B., Marsh P., Dvorchak, P. A., Groessl, E. K., et al. (1997). An exploratory study of male recovering substance abusers living in a self-help, self-governed setting. *Journal of Mental Health Administration, 24*, 332–339.

Kim, K. L., Davis, M. I., Jason, L. A., & Ferrari, J. R. (2006). Structural social support: Impact on adult substance use and recovery attempts. *Journal of Prevention & Intervention in the Community, 31*, 85–94.

McGrath, J. E. (1984). *Groups: Interaction and performance.* Englewood Cliffs, NJ: Prentice-Hall.

McMillan, D. W., & Chavis, D. M. (1986). Sense of community: A definition and theory. *American Journal of Community Psychology, 14*, 6–23.

Oakes, M. E. (2003). Differences in judgments of food healthfulness by young and elderly women. *Food Quality and Preference, 14*, 227–236.

Oxford House, Inc. (n.d.). Retrieved December 21, 2006, from http://www.oxfordhouse.org

Proescholdbell, R. J., & Roosa, M. W. (2005, June). *Concepts for the design of psychological sense of community interventions.* Poster presentation, Society for Community Research and Action, Urbana, Illinois.

Prosper, V., Sherman, S. R., & Howe, J. L. (2004). Living arrangements for older New Yorkers. In Project 2015: The Future of Aging in New York State. New York State Office for the Aging. Retrieved December 21, 2007, from http://www.aging.state.ny.us/explore/project2015

Sarason, S. B. (1974). *The psychological sense of community: Prospects for a community psychology.* San Francisco: Jossey-Bass.

Skajaeveland, O., Garling, T., & Maeland, J. G. (1996). A multidimensional measure of neighborhoods. *American Journal of Community Psychology, 24*, 413–435.

Abstinence Social Support: The Impact of Children in Oxford House

EMILY ORTIZ, BA, JOSEFINA ALVAREZ, PhD,
LEONARD A. JASON, PhD, JOSEPH R. FERRARI, PhD, and
DAVID R. GROH, PhD

DePaul University

The present study compared the characteristics of individuals living with (42 men, 52 women) and without children (561 men, 241 women) residing in a communal-living recovery program called Oxford Houses. Results indicated that men living with children and women living without children had more general social support, compared to men living without children and women living with children. Additionally, women and residents of adult-only houses reported having more drug users in their social networks. However, men and women living with and without children reported similar levels of social support for abstinence. It is suggested that that men in recovery who take care of their children are in situations more advantageous to sustained recovery and have more resources compared to recovering women with children. Women in substance abuse recovery and taking care of children may require additional resources and assistance compared to men.

Substance-related disorders are most prevalent during young adulthood, and approximately half of substance-abusing individuals who seek treatment are parents (McMahon, Winkel, Luthar, & Rounsaville, 2005; Meier, Donmall, & McElduff, 2004; Stewart, Gossop, & Trakada, 2007). However, researchers generally neglected the experiences of substance-using parents and their

Funding was made possible in part through National Institute on Drug Abuse (NIDA) grants #5F31DA16037 and #R01DA13231.

children (Suchman & Luthar, 2002). Research on parenting among men who abuse substances has been particularly rare (McMahon et al., 2005).

The presence of children is often thought to add an extra burden to individuals in recovery, and recovering women in particular. Substance-related disorders are more prevalent among men; thus, more men than women in recovery report being parents (McMahon et al., 2005). However, a greater proportion of women seeking substance abuse services are parents, and women in recovery are more likely to have custody of their children (McMahon et al., 2005; Meier et al., 2004; Stewart et al., 2007). Nonetheless, these women are less likely than men to be supported throughout treatment (Reed, 1985). In many cases, alternative child care is too expensive or simply not available to women, especially those with lower socioeconomic status, and few substance abuse treatment programs provide child care options or allow children into the program (Nelson-Zlupko, Kauffman, & More, 1995). Furthermore, addicted women are frequently discouraged by family members from seeking treatment due to the concern that treatment could interfere with caring for their family (Nelson-Zlupko et al.).

Studies indicated that children may provide added motivation to stop using and may serve as sources of support for abstinence (Luthar, D'Avanzo, & Hites, 2003; McMahon, Winkel, Suchman, & Luthar, 2001). Christensen (1999) found that children of alcoholic parents frequently provide specific social support for abstinence through attempting, generally unsuccessfully, to convince their parents to quit drinking. Koski-Jännes (1991) suggested that the relationship between having children and reduced drinking results from the social support provided by the children A child's response to his or her parent's sobriety may provide more meaningful social support than that of the spouse or other adults (Koski-Jännes). Finally, children were cited by parents in recovery as the number one relationship that helped them decide to enter treatment (Mays, Beckman, Oranchak, & Harper, 1994).

In addition, parents often receive outside social pressures discouraging substance use. For example, only 3% of Ontario adults in 1992 felt that it was acceptable for parents to drink enough to be slightly intoxicated in front of their children, and 53% felt that consuming alcohol in front of children is never appropriate (Ferris, Templeton, & Wong, 1994). Gullestad (1984) found that blue-collar mothers in Bergen who were young and generally divorced received great pressure from their neighbors to abstain. Additionally, the recent push to avoid drinking during pregnancy may provide additional pressure for abstinence among parents, especially mothers (Room, 1996).

In recent years, substance abuse treatment programs addressed the needs of recovering mothers by including children in both residential and outpatient interventions (Dawe, Harnett, Rendalls, & Staiger, 2003; Knight, Hood, Logan, & Chatham, 1999; Wexler, Cuadrado, & Stevens, 1998; Wobie, Eyler, Conlon, & Clarke, 1997; Worley, Conners, Crone, Williams, & Bokony, 2005). These programs provided a variety of services, including parenting education and child-focused interventions. A number of studies indicate that including children in their mothers' treatment leads to better retention and outcome among women in recovery (Conners, Grant, Crone, & Whiteside-Mansell, 2006; Hughes, Coletti, Neri, Urmann, Stahl, Sicilian, et al., 1995; Stevens & Patton, 1998; Szuster, Rich, Chung, & Bisconer, 1996).

In addition, having children may relate to greater success in substance abuse treatment. A Finnish study (Koski-Jännes, 1991) found that compared to women without children, those who had children tended to have more days abstinent before treatment, stay in treatment longer, and have greater treatment compliance. In fact, living with children was the strongest predictor of recovery in their study, even stronger than the number of children or having a partner (Koski-Jännes).

An example of a supportive community-based recovery home for individuals dealing with substance abuse problems is Oxford House (OH; see Jason, Ferrari, Davis, & Olson, 2006). A low cost, self-run, democratic recovery home model, Oxford House has grown since 1975 to over 1,200 homes across the USA, 30 in Canada, and 8 in Australia. Regarding the operation and maintenance of Oxford Houses, no professional staff is involved, enabling residents to create their own rules for communal governance. Residents live together in a democratic, single-sex home and provide each other with a supportive abstinent mutual-support network. The residents are allowed to stay indefinitely, provided that they pay rent, abstain from alcohol and drug use, and avoid disruptive behavior. Failure to comply with these guidelines is grounds for expulsion from the house.

Regarding parenting practices, Oxford Houses are single-sex dwellings, and a number of houses allow mothers and fathers to live with their minor children (Oxford House, 2003). Fathers—or, more typically, mothers—live in an Oxford House with one or more of their children along with other residents who have no children in the house. For example, in northern Illinois, eight women on average live in a house, and up to four of those women may have children with them. This arrangement allows for greater financial stability and prevents overcrowding (Paul Molloy, personal communication, December, 2006). The other house residents are expected to take an active role in helping take care of the children in the house. Oxford House also generally requires mothers to take some form of parenting class outside of the houses.

Several research studies have focused specifically on parents and children within Oxford Houses. Multiple studies demonstrated that the children in Oxford House have a positive effect on the recovery of the adult women residents (d'Arlach, Olson, Jason, & Ferrari, 2006; Kim, Davis, Jason, & Ferrari, 2006). This positive effect was identical for both mothers and nonmothers, possibly because having children present leads to increased responsibility among all house residents, aiding in recovery (d'Arlach et al., 2006). These women also reported experiencing a high sense of satisfaction with the houses and stated that residents provided one another with support for abstinence and parenting. Finally, while there are several Oxford Houses for fathers with children, the experience of these male residents has not been studied.

Social support plays a significant role in the effectiveness of Oxford House (Groh, Jason, Davis, Olson, & Ferrari, 2007; Jason, Davis, Ferrari, & Anderson, 2007). Regarding general social support, Oxford House residents rated "fellowship with similar peers" the most important aspect of living in an Oxford House (Jason, Ferrari, Dvorchak, Groessl, & Molloy, 1997). Oxford House also provides residents with abstinence-specific social support networks consisting of other residents in recovery (Flynn, Alvarez, Jason, Olson, Ferrari, & Davis, 2006). Longer lengths of stay in Oxford House related to less support for substance use (Davis & Jason, 2005) and increased support for abstinence (Majer, Jason, Ferrari, Venable, & Olson, 2002). Furthermore, Oxford House residents whose social networks provided less support for substance use were more likely to remain abstinent (Jason et al., 2007). Other studies report that women who have supportive relationships are more likely to complete substance abuse treatment and have better outcomes (Coughey, Feighan, Cheney, & Klein, 1998; Knight et al., 1999). Finally, abstinence-specific social support has been found to be a particularly strong predictor of long-term abstinence following treatment (Longabaugh, Wirtz, Beattie, Noel, & Stout, 1995; Longabaugh, Wirtz, Zweben, & Stout, 1999).

The current study explored the experiences of different types of general and substance use-specific support among men and women living with and without children in Oxford House. Based on research indicating that mothers have better outcomes when living with their children during substance abuse treatment, we hypothesized that both men and women living in Oxford Houses with children would experience more general social support and more support for remaining abstinent than men and women living without children in Oxford House.

METHODS

Procedure

Analysis of data provided by Oxford House using a geographic information systems (GIS) program indicated that houses clustered in the states of Washington, Oregon, Pennsylvania, New Jersey, North Carolina, Illinois, and Texas. Participants were recruited either by research staff who visited 170 Oxford Houses in these states or at the 2001 Oxford House World Convention. After explaining the study to participants and securing informed consent, research assistants administered the study's measures in a group format. Research assistants were available to answer questions while participants completed the paper and pencil measures (see Jason et al., 2007). The current

TABLE 1 Mean Demographics for Men and Women Living With and Without Children

Descriptor Variables	Children	No Children
Age:		
Males	40.85	39.23
Females	34.50	36.89
Monthly Income:		
Males	1267.62	1078.61
Females	538.79	792.22
Education (years):		
Males	12.78	12.75
Females	12.26	12.39
Length of Stay in OH (years):		
Males	1.86	.925
Females	.723	.718

investigation reports baseline data for the longitudinal study, which collected data every 4 months for a period of approximately 1 year (Jason et al.).

Participants

Participants included 42 men and 52 women living in Oxford Houses with children and 561 men and 241 women living in houses without children. Participant demographic characteristics are presented in Table 1. Among participants residing in houses with children, 52 (55%) were from Washington or Oregon, 24 (26%) resided in houses in Pennsylvania or New Jersey, 12 (13%) lived in the Midwest or Texas, and 6 (6%) resided in North Carolina. Among participants living in houses with no children, 280 (34%) lived in North Carolina, 190 (24%) resided in Washington or Oregon, 168 (21%) lived in the Northeast, and 165 (21%) lived in the Midwest or Texas.

In terms of ethnicity, 62 (66%) participants living in houses with children were European Americans, whereas 18 (19%) were African Americans, 3 (3%) were Hispanics/Latinos, and 11 (12%) represented other ethnicities including Asian Americans, American Indians, and biracial or multiracial individuals. Among participants living in houses without children, 462 (58%) were European Americans, 287 (36%) were African Americans, 28 (3%) were Hispanics/Latinos, and 26 (3%) represented other ethnicities. Approximately 50% of participants in both types of houses were never married; 45% were divorced, separated, or widowed; and 5% were married.

ANOVAs were run to test differences in age, years of education, monthly income, and time in Oxford House at baseline. A significant main effect for gender, $F(1,890) = 18.35$, $p < .001$, and a significant interaction between gender and house type, $F(1,890) = 3.87$, $p < .05$, was found for participants' age. A significant main effect for gender, $F(1,868) = 3.91$, $p < .05$, was found for years of education. ANCOVAs, controlling for years of education, indicated a significant main effect for gender, $F(1,842) = 25.13, p < .001$, and a significant interaction between gender and house type, $F(1,842) = 4.31$, $p < .05$, for monthly income. A significant main effect for gender, $F(1,884) = 24.02, p < .001$, and house type, $F(1,884) = 11.48, p < .001$, was found for time in Oxford House. The interaction between gender and house type also was significant, $F(1,884) = 11.20, p < .001$, for time in Oxford House at baseline.

Measures

Participants completed the Addiction Severity Index—Lite (ASI; McLellan, Kushner, Metzger, Peters, Smith, Grissom, et al., 1992), a valid and reliable measure of lifetime and recent substance use and related medical, psychological, family, employment, and legal problems. The ASI collected demographic and treatment history data and provided seven valid and reliable composite scores (i.e., drug, alcohol, medical, psychological, family, legal, and employment) based on reports of problems during the 30 days prior to scale administration. In the current study, the ASI was used to collect demographic data.

Finally, a modified version of the Important People and Activities Inventory (IPA; Clifford & Longabaugh, 1991) with the activities items omitted (i.e., the IP) was administered to assess social support variables. Additionally, the modified version of this measure administered for the current study included questions regarding alcohol as well as illicit drug use. The IP requires respondents to identify important members in their networks with whom they have had frequent contact within the past 6 months. For each person the participant lists in his or her network, the scale examines the type of relationship (e.g., spouse, parent, or friend), the duration of relationship in years, and the frequency of contact. In addition, the participant reports how often the network member drinks, how much the network member drinks on a maximum drinking day, and the network member's overall drinking status (i.e., heavy, moderate, light, abstainer, or recovering). The IP was used in several studies including Project MATCH and demonstrated good test–retest reliability and construct validity (Beattie, Longabaugh, Elliott, Stout, Fava, & Noel, 1993; Longabaugh et al., 1995, 1998). The current study scored the IP according to the three factors derived by Groh and his colleagues: general social support, drinking behaviors of network members, and support for drinking from network members (Groh, Olson, Jason, Ferrari, & Davis, in press). Higher scores on the IP indicate greater support for substance use.

RESULTS

Differences in general social support between men and women living in Oxford Houses with and without children were examined using an ANOVA. Distributions for drinking behaviors of network members and support for substance use among network members were skewed. Therefore, these scores were dichotomized into "high" and "low" based on a median split and analyzed using chi-square analyses.

In terms of general social support, a significant interaction was found between house type and gender, $F(1, 896) = 9.89$, $p < .001$, such that men living in houses with children and women living in houses without children had higher levels of general social support compared to men living without children and women living with children. Chi-squares found no significant association between gender or house type and drinking behaviors of network members. However, a significant association was found between the illicit drug use behaviors of network members and both gender, X^2 (1, 871) = 12.25, $p < .001$, and house type, X^2 (1, 871) = 3.87, $p < .05$, such that women and residents of houses without children had more individuals who used illicit drugs in their social networks. No significant association was found between gender or house type and support for drinking or illicit drug use.

DISCUSSION

This study explored demographic and social support differences among men and women living in Oxford Houses with and without children at the baseline of a longitudinal, national study of Oxford House residents. Results indicated a number of important between-group differences that may have implications for recovery. For instance, men were significantly older than women. Although women with children comprised the youngest group of participants, men with children were the oldest group. Men had significantly more years of education than women along with higher incomes, even after controlling for years of education. Furthermore, women with children had the lowest whereas men with children had the highest incomes of all groups. These differences are important because age, education, and employment status have been found to predict recovery outcomes (Brewer, Catalano, Haggerty, Gainey, & Fleming, 1998; Scott-Lennox, Rose, Bohlig, & Lennox, 2000). Significant gender and house type differences were also found in terms of time in Oxford House: men living in Oxford Houses with children had stays that were over twice as long as those of the other groups. All of the findings indicate a number of advantages for men compared to women living in Oxford Houses with children.

Analysis of baseline social support data indicated that men living in Oxford Houses *with children* and women living in houses *without children* had more general social support that men living without children and women living with children. This is consistent with past research suggesting that women are less likely than men to be supported throughout treatment (Reed, 1985) and that women are often discouraged by from seeking treatment because it might interfere with child care (Nelson-Zlupko et al., 1995). However, no significant group differences were found in terms of abstinence-specific social support for either alcohol or illicit drug use. In terms of the composition of social support networks, no group differences were found regarding the alcohol use habits of friends and family members. However, results indicated that women and residents of Oxford Houses without children had more illicit drug users in their social networks. Thus, having children may help protect against maintaining relationships with negative drug-using friends and family members. However, these findings are partially in contrast to research suggesting that compared to men, recovering women with children might have more abstinence support in their social networks (Room, 1996), which can include avoiding friends and family who use drugs.

In summary, the results of this investigation suggests that men in recovery who take care of their children are in situations more conducive to sustained recovery and have more resources (i.e., they are older, are more educated, have higher incomes, and have longer lengths of stay in OH), including positive social supports (i.e., they receive more general support and have fewer drug users in their social networks), whereas women in recovery who take care of their children have the least of these types of resources. It is possible that recovering women who have children are frequently forced to take care of their children because no one else is available to take on these child care duties; on the other hand, recovering men may be more likely to take care of their children when they are doing well in recovery and elect to take on this responsibility. Therefore, it is suggested that recovering women taking care of children may require additional resources compared to recovering men taking care of children. It may be important for the Oxford House organization to provide more assistance when opening homes for women with children. In addition, clinicians and treatment providers working with women in recovery with children may want to address these additional struggles and help these individuals develop supportive social networks.

REFERENCES

Beattie, M. C., Longabaugh R., Elliott G., Stout, R. L., Fava J., & Noel, N. E. (1993). Effect of the social environment on alcohol involvement and subjective well-being prior to alcoholism treatment. *Journal of Studies on Alcohol, 54,* 283–296.

Brewer, D. D., Catalano, R. F., Haggerty, K. H., Gainey, R. R., & Fleming, C. B. (1998). A meta-analysis of predictors of continued drug use during and after treatment for opiate addiction. *Addiction, 93*, 73–92.

Christensen, E. (1999). Aspects of a preventive approach to support children of alcoholics. *Child Abuse Review, 6*, 24–34.

Clifford, P. R., & Longabaugh, R. (1991). *Manual for the administration of the Important People and Activities instrument: Project MATCH.* Providence, RI: Center for Alcohol and Addiction Studies, Brown University.

Conners, N. A., Grant, A., Crone, C. C., & Whiteside-Mansell, L. (2006). Substance abuse treatment for mothers: Treatment outcomes and the impact of length of stay. *Journal of Substance Abuse Treatment, 31*, 447–456.

Coughey, K., Feighan, K., Cheney, R., & Klein, G. (1998). Retention in an aftercare program for recovering women. *Substance Use & Misuse, 33*, 917–933.

d'Arlach, L., Olson, B. D., Jason, L. A., & Ferrari, J. R. (2006). Children, women, and substance abuse: A look at recovery in a communal setting. *Journal of Prevention & Intervention in the Community, 31*, 121–132.

Davis, M. I., & Jason, L. A. (2005). Sex differences in social support and self-efficacy within a recovery community. *American Journal of Community Psychology, 36*, 259–274.

Dawe, S., Harnett, P. H., Rendalls, V., & Staiger, P. (2003). Improving family functioning and child outcome in methadone maintained families: The Parents under Pressure programme. *Drug and Alcohol Review, 22*, 299–307.

Ferris, J., Templeton, L., & Wong, S. (1994). Alcohol, tobacco and marijuana use, norms, problems and policy attitudes among Ontario adults. Toronto: Addiction Research Foundation, Internal Document No. 118.

Flynn, A. M., Alvarez, J., Jason, L. A., Olson, B. D., Ferrari, J. R., & Davis, M. I. (2006). African American Oxford House residents: Sources of abstinent social networks. *Journal of Prevention and Intervention in the Community, 31*, 111–119.

Groh, D. R., Jason, L. A., Davis, M. I., Olson, B. D., & Ferrari, J. R. (2007). Friends, family, and alcohol abuse: An examination of general and alcohol-specific social support. *The American Journal on Addictions, 16*, 49–55.

Groh, D. R., Olson, B. D., Jason, L. A., Ferrari, J. R., & Davis, M. I. (in press). A factor analysis of the Important People Inventory. *Alcohol & Alcoholism.* Advance Access published May 25, 2007. doi:10.1093/alcalc/agm012

Gullestad, M. (1984). Kitchen-table society. Oslo: Universitetsforlaget.

Hughes, P. H., Coletti, S. D., Neri, R. L., Urmann, C. F., Stahl, S., Sicilian, D. M., et al (1995). Retaining cocaine-abusing women in a therapeutic community: The effect of a child live-in program. *American Journal of Public Health, 85*, 1149–1152.

Jason, L. A., Davis, M. I., Ferrari, J. R., & Anderson, E. (2007). The need for substance abuse after-care: A longitudinal analysis of Oxford House. *Addictive Behaviors, 32*, 808–813.

Jason, L. A., Ferrari, J. R., Davis, M. I., & Olson, B. D. (2006). *Creating communities for addiction recovery: The Oxford House model.* Binghamton, NY: Haworth Press.

Jason, L. A., Ferrari, J. R., Dvorchak, P. A., Groessl, E. J., & Molloy, J. P. (1997). The characteristics of alcoholics in self-help residential treatment settings: A multi-site study of Oxford House. *Alcoholism Treatment Quarterly*, *15*, 53–63.

Kim, K. L., Davis, M. I., Jason, L. A., & Ferrari, J. R. (2006). Structural social support: Impact on adult substance use and recovery attempts. *Journal of Prevention & Intervention in the Community*, *31*, 85–94.

Knight, D. K., Hood, P. E., Logan, S. M., & Chatham, L. R. (1999). Residential treatment for women with dependent children: One agency's approach. *Journal of Psychoactive Drugs*, *31*, 339–351.

Koski-Jännes, A. (1991). The role of children in the recovery of alcoholic clients. *Contemporary Drug Problems*, *18*, 629–644.

Longabaugh, R., Wirtz, P., Beattie, M., Noel, N., & Stout, R. (1995). Matching treatment focus to patient social investment and support: 18 month follow-up results. *Journal of Consulting and Clinical Psychology*, *63*, 296–307.

Longabaugh, R., Wirtz, P. W., Zweben, A., & Stout, R. L. (1998). Network support for drinking, Alcoholics Anonymous and long-term matching effects. *Addiction*, *93*, 1313–1333.

Luthar, S. S., D'Avanzo, K., & Hites, S. (2003). Maternal drug abuse versus other psychological disturbances. In S. S. Luthar (Ed.), *Resilience and vulnerability: Adaptation in the context of childhood adversities* (pp. 104–129). New York: Cambridge University Press.

Majer, J. M., Jason, L. A., Ferrari, J. R., Venable, L. B., & Olson, D. D. (2002). Social support and self-efficacy for abstinence: Is peer identification an issue? *Journal of Substance Abuse Treatment*, *23*, 209–215.

Mays, V. M., Beckman, L. J., Oranchak, E., & Harper, B. (1994). Perceived social support for help-seeking behaviors of Black heterosexual and homosexually active women alcoholics. *Psychology of Addictive Behaviors*, *8*, 235–242.

McLellan, A. T., Kushner, H., Metzger, D., Peters, R., Smith, I., Grissom, G., et al. (1992). The fifth edition of the Addiction Severity Index. *Journal of Substance Abuse Treatment*, *9*, 199–213.

McMahon, T. J., Winkel, J., Suchman, N., & Luthar, S. S. (2001). Drug dependence, parenting responsibility, and treatment history: Why doesn't mom go for help? *Drug and Alcohol Dependence*, *65*, 105–114.

McMahon, T. J., Winkel, J., Luthar, S. S., & Rounsaville, B. J. (2005). Looking for Poppa: Parenting status of men versus women seeking drug abuse treatment. *The American Journal of Drug and Alcohol Abuse*, *1*, 79–91.

Meier, P. S., Donmall, M. C., & McElduff, P. (2004). Characteristics of drug users who do or do not have care of their children. *Addiction*, *99*, 955–961.

Nelson-Zlupko, L., Kauffman, E., & More, M. M. (1995). Gender differences in drug addiction and treatment: Implications for social work intervention with substance-abusing women. *Social Work*, *40*, 45–54.

Oxford House. (2003). *Oxford House manual*. Retrieved December 2, 2006, from http://www.oxfordhouse.org

Reed, B. G. (1985). Drug misuse and dependency in women: The meaning and implications of being considered a special population or minority group. *International Journal of the Addictions*, *20*, 13–62.

Room, R. (1996). Gender roles and interactions in drinking and drug use. *Journal of Substance Abuse*, *8*, 227–239.

Scott-Lennox, J., Rose, R., Bohlig, A., & Lennox, R. J. (2000). The impact of women's family status on completion of substance abuse treatment. *Behavioral Health Services Research, 27*, 366–379.

Stewart, D., Gossop, M., & Trakada, K. (2007). Drug dependent parents: Childcare responsibilities, involvement with treatment services, and treatment outcomes. *Addictive Behaviors, 32*, 1657–1668.

Stevens, S. J., & Patton, T. (1998). Residential treatment for drug addicted women and their children: Effective treatment strategies. *Drugs & Society, 13*, 235–249.

Suchman, N. E., & Luthar, S. S. (2000). Maternal addiction, child maladjustment, and socio-demographic risks: Implication for parenting behaviors. *Addiction, 95*, 1417–1428.

Szuster, R. R., Rich, L. L., Chung, A., & Bisconer, S. W. (1996). Treatment retention in women's residential chemical dependency treatment: The effect of admission with children. *Substance Use & Misuse, 31*, 1001–1013.

Wexler, H. K., Cuadrado, M., & Stevens, S. J. (1998). Residential treatment for women: Behavioral and psychological outcomes. *Drugs & Society, 13*, 213–233.

Wobie, K., Eyler, F. D., Conlon, M., & Clarke, L. (1997). Women and children in residential treatment: Outcomes for mothers and their infants. *Journal of Drug Issues, 27*, 585–606.

Worley, L. M., Conners, N. A., Crone, C. C., Williams, V. L., & Bokony, P. A. (2005). Building a residential treatment program for dually diagnosed women with their children. *Archives of Women's Mental Health, 8*, 105–111.

A Longitudinal Analysis of Criminal and Aggressive Behaviors Among a National Sample of Adults in Mutual-Help Recovery Homes

DARRIN M. AASE, MA, and LEONARD A. JASON, PhD

Center for Community Research, DePaul University

BRADLEY D. OLSON, PhD

Foley Center for the Study of Lives, Northwestern University

JOHN M. MAJER, PhD

Department of Social Sciences, Richard J. Daley College

JOSEPH R. FERRARI, PhD

Department of Psychology, DePaul University

MARGARET I. DAVIS, PhD

Department of Psychology, Dickinson College

SANDRA M. VIRTUE, PhD

Department of Psychology, DePaul University

Criminal and aggressive behaviors are frequently observed among those recovering from substance abuse problems. In the present one-year longitudinal study, a national sample of residents from self-governed, communal-living recovery homes for substance abuse completed baseline and follow-up measures of criminal and aggressive behavior. Results indicated that a length of stay of 6 months or longer was associated with lower levels of self-reported criminal and aggressive behaviors at the one-year follow-up. Environmental mechanisms proposed as influences for these outcomes, as well as treatment implications, are discussed.

Portions of this article were based on the master's thesis of the first author. This research was financially supported by the U.S. National Institute on Drug Abuse (grant number DA13231).

Although substance use and its correlates have been thoroughly investigated, less is known about the role of aggression and criminal behavior during recovery. Behavioral problems such as aggression and criminal activity frequently co-occur with substance use (Eklund & Klinteberg, 2005; Thomson, 1999). For example, over 40% of offenders on probation or in local U.S. jails were found to be drinking at the time of their offense (Bureau of Justice Statistics [BJS], 1998). While less than 10% of the general population has a substance use disorder, 68% of jailed inmates meet diagnostic criteria (BJS, 2005). Additionally, 90% of crack or cocaine users reported a history of crime that involved theft or selling drugs (Inciardi, McBride, McCoy, & Chitwood, 1994).

Furthermore, both alcohol and drug use have been frequently associated with domestic violence (e.g., Murphy, Winters, O'Farrell, Fals-Stewart, & Murphy, 2005) and other aggressive acts (Bushman & Cooper, 1990; Miller & Potter-Efron, 1989). Alcohol and drug use may lead to reduced inhibition of these behaviors, while involvement in deviant activities might facilitate the development of substance abuse through social learning mechanisms (Kaplan, 1995). This reciprocal relationship between substance use and externalizing behaviors presents difficulties for the treatment of both issues. Consequently, interventions that address both types of behavior might be more effective than interventions that focus on one issue (e.g., Putt, Dowd, & McCormick, 2001).

An innovative setting that might address criminal and violent behavior problems in a cost-effective manner is Oxford House, a network of over 1,200 self-governing, mutual-help recovery homes for individuals in recovery (Jason, Davis, Ferrari, & Bishop, 2001). The Oxford House model consists of self-run, democratic communities that do not include professional staff. There also are no restrictions on how long a person can remain a resident (Oxford House, 2000). By combining elements of residential treatment and mutual-help organizations, Oxford Houses might function as continuous sources of mutual support for individuals in recovery (Olson, Jason, Ferrari, & Hutcheson, 2005).

Individuals in recovery with aggressive or criminal behavior problems might respond favorably to the structure provided by Oxford House. For example, Ferrari, Jason, Davis, Olson, and Alvarez (2004) compared rules and regulations between traditional therapeutic communities and Oxford Houses, finding that Oxford Houses provided more strict rules related to disruptive behavior between residents and more regulations involving house living. However, they also found that Oxford Houses permit more personal liberties for residents compared to therapeutic communities, which might reduce noncompliance and rebellious attitudes toward strict behavior codes (Ferrari et al., 2004).

A recent study of the Oxford House model examined individuals randomly assigned to either regular aftercare or to an Oxford House upon discharge from inpatient substance abuse treatment (Jason, Olson, Ferrari, & Lo Sasso, 2006). Oxford House residents had significantly better outcomes for both substance use and incarceration rates when compared to participants in the usual care condition. A study of the same sample found better treatment outcomes for self-regulation, substance use, and incarceration when Oxford House residents stayed for at least 6 months (Jason, Olson, Ferrari, Majer, Alvarez, & Stout, 2007). A recent study of a national sample of Oxford House residents found that staying in an Oxford House for 6 months or longer predicted higher rates of abstinence from substance use (Jason, Davis, Ferrari, & Anderson, 2007). Researchers studying other residential treatment modalities for substance abuse have also found that a 6-month length of stay is a critical time-point that is associated with better outcomes for abstinence, illegal activity, and employment (Bleiberg, Devlin, Croan, & Briscoe, 1994; Hubbard, Craddock, Flynn, Anderson, & Etheridge, 1997).

Given the connection between aggressive and criminal behaviors and substance abuse, the present study expands upon the work of Jason, Davis, et al. (2007) by examining these behaviors over time in the same national sample of Oxford House residents. The present study examined a subset of this sample of Oxford House residents and measured their self-reported criminal and aggressive behaviors for one year. It was specifically predicted that individuals who remained in an Oxford House for at least 6 months after the baseline assessment would have better outcomes on measures of both criminal and aggressive behaviors at a one-year follow-up.

METHOD

Participants

A total of 897 participants (293 females, 604 males) were recruited to be in a national study on Oxford House residents (for a more detailed discussion of these recruitment methods, see Jason, Davis, et al., 2007). Prior to a baseline assessment, the full sample of participants spent an average of 10.9 months ($SD = 15.05$) with a range of a few days to 10.2 years living in one of 170 Oxford Houses located across the United States. However, because we were interested in examining length of residence in an Oxford House prospectively, the present study examined a subset of the national sample ($n = 165$) who lived in an Oxford House for 30 days or less prior to the baseline assessment. These participants were unique within the sample because they did not have extensive experience within an Oxford House, which provided an opportunity to explore potential effects of living in an Oxford House over time. Of these participants, 88 (35 females, 53 males) completed all of the baseline and one-year follow-up measures, and constitute the subsample in the analysis.

The average age of the subsample was 36.4 ($SD = 8.1$, range $= 18.6$–55.7 years) and their average number of years of education was 12.6 ($SD = 1.8$). The subsample consisted of 58.0% Caucasians, 33.0% African Americans, 5.7% Hispanic/Latinos, and 3.4% other ethnicities. Employment characteristics of the sample were assessed, and 62.5% of the participants were employed full time, 15.9% were employed part time, and 21.6% were unemployed. In the subsample, 53.4% reported being single; 40.9% were divorced, widowed, or separated; and 3.4% reported being married. Average monthly income for residents was $610.02 ($SD = \$682.96$). With regard to legal status, 13.6% were currently awaiting legal charges. The authors believe that this is a representative sample of individuals in recovery for substance use.

Procedure

Approval from the Institutional Review Board was obtained prior to the study, and interviewers were provided with training on administering the surveys. After recruitment, all participants were informed that their answers would remain completely confidential and that they were allowed to withdraw from the study at any time. At baseline, the research personnel discussed the consent form with participants and asked them to complete a telephone contact sheet for reaching them at follow-up waves of the study. The majority of surveys were administered to participants in their houses or at the 2001 Oxford House World Convention. Participants who were recruited at the convention completed the survey in a conference room that had been set aside for that purpose (see Jason, Davis et al., 2007). The research personnel went over the directions and remained available to answer questions. After completing the surveys, participants received a $15 payment.

The study contained four waves of assessment, with data collected in 4-month intervals. For all waves after baseline, research personnel attempted to contact participants based on the telephone contact information they provided. Once contacted, all other assessment waves included surveys administered either in person, by mail, or over the telephone, and participants were again given a $15 payment for each wave. All participants were thanked for volunteering to participate and given the research team's contact information if they had questions. After all of the data was collected, all participants were given written educational feedback that discussed the success of the study and restated the purpose of the project.

Measures

General baseline demographic and background information for participants, including initial time living in an Oxford House, was obtained from self-report items on the Addiction Severity Index—Lite (ASI; McLellan, Kushner,

Metzger, Peters, Smith, Grissom, et al., 1992). The ASI examines several areas commonly affected by substance abuse, such as medical condition, illegal activity, employment, family relations, and psychiatric condition. This measure is widely used and has test–retest reliability of .83 or higher (McLellan et al., 1992).

Time in an Oxford House was determined using Miller and Del Boca's (1994) Form 90 at each subsequent assessment. Adequate to excellent test–retest reliabilities have been reported for alcohol consumption (0.91 to 0.97) and days living in a residence (0.74 to 0.99; Miller, 1996). Consistent with Jason, Davis et al. (2007), this information from all follow-up waves was used to create a dichotomous variable for whether or not each participant remained living in an Oxford House for 6 months or not throughout the course of the study.

The *Global Appraisal of Individual Needs—Quick Screen* (*GAIN-QS*; Titus & Dennis, 2000) was used to measure criminal and aggressive behavior. This is a clinical screening instrument assessing a variety of psychological issues among the general population (Titus & Dennis, 2000). For determining criminal and aggressive behaviors in the current study, two specific subscales were used: The *General Crime Index* (*GCI*), a four-item measure of self-reported illegal activities over the past twelve months (original $M = 0.44$, $SD = 0.89$, $\alpha = 0.69$), and the *Conduct Disorder-Aggression Index* (*CDAI*), a six-item measure of aggressive and disruptive behaviors (original $M = 2.01$, $SD = 1.87$, $\alpha = 0.78$; Titus & Dennis, 2000). In the current subsample, the GCI had a baseline mean score of .98 ($SD = 1.29$; $\alpha = 0.75$), and the CDAI had a baseline mean score of 2.6 ($SD = 1.90$; $\alpha = 0.79$).

RESULTS

Group Comparisons

Chi square analyses and independent samples *t*-tests were used to compare groups prior to the analysis. The group that remained in the study and the attrition group did not differ based on a number of variables: baseline crime and aggression scores, gender, ethnicity, marital status, whether they were presently awaiting legal charges, parole or probation status, employment status, total monthly income, years of education, lifetime incarceration in months, length of sobriety, income, age, and years of education.

Within the subsample of 88 participants, 41 stayed in an Oxford House for 6 months or longer. These residents were compared to those who left prior to 6 months ($n = 47$). The two groups did not differ significantly based on the following variables: baseline crime and aggression scores, ethnicity, marital status, whether they were presently awaiting legal charges, parole or probation status, employment status, total monthly income, years of education, length of sobriety, income, age, and years of education. However, the group that stayed in an Oxford house for 6 months or longer was more likely to be male, χ^2 (1, $N = 88$) = 5.37, $p < .05$, and had fewer lifetime months of incarceration, $t(86) = 2.0$, $p = .049$. These variables were analyzed in relation to the outcome variables, and no significant associations were found. Therefore, we excluded these variables from the analyses.

Longitudinal Analyses

SPSS GLM was used to conduct two univariate ANCOVAs comparing the groups based on their length of residence in an Oxford House on criminal and aggressive behavior outcomes. Because the groups based on time in an Oxford House did not significantly differ on baseline scores for criminal or aggressive behavior, ANCOVA is more powerful than using a repeated measures approach (Weinfurt, 2000, p. 341). Baseline scores for crime and aggression were used as covariates in the analyses, and follow-up scores were the dependent variables.

For criminal behavior, there was a main effect of staying in an Oxford House for 6 months or longer, $F(1, 85) = 7.88$, $p = .006$. An examination of the estimated marginal means indicated that when controlling for baseline criminal behavior scores, those who remained in an Oxford House for 6 months or longer had significantly lower ($M = 0.20$, $SE = 0.13$) follow-up crime scores than those who left prior to 6 months ($M = 0.68$, $SE = 0.12$). With regard to aggressive behavior, the baseline aggression score covariate was significant in predicting follow-up aggression, $F(1, 85) = 4.72$, $p = .033$. Furthermore, there was a main effect of staying in an Oxford House for 6 months or longer, $F(1, 85) = 4.83$, $p = .031$. When controlling for baseline aggression scores, those who remained in an Oxford House for 6 months or longer had significantly lower ($M = 1.34$, $SE = 0.23$) follow-up aggressive behavior scores than those who left prior to 6 months ($M = 2.02$, $SE = 0.21$).

DISCUSSION

This study examined the impact of time living in an Oxford House on self-reported criminal and aggressive behaviors. It was predicted that Oxford House residents who continued residence for at least 6 months in an Oxford House would have lower scores on subscales measuring these behaviors than residents who did not remain in Oxford House for 6 months. When examining these behavioral outcomes over time, staying in an Oxford House for 6 months or longer was associated with lower scores on measures of both criminal and aggressive behaviors.

There are several potential reasons why longer residency in an Oxford House might be associated with reduced criminal behavior. From a practical perspective, Oxford Houses tend to be in neighborhoods where there is low drug trafficking and criminal activity (Jason et al., 2001; Ferrari, Jason, Blake, Davis, & Olson, 2006), thereby reducing opportunities to become involved in illegal activities. Additionally, most Oxford House residents are able to maintain stable employment and an adequate income (Jason, Ferrari, Smith, Marsh, Dvorchak, Groessl, et al., 1997). In fact, Jason et al. (2006) found that Oxford House residents had a significantly higher monthly income at a 2-year follow-up than individuals who received standard substance abuse treatment.

In addition, the results of the present study supported our prediction that more time in an Oxford House would be associated with lower aggression scores. This outcome is consistent with previous research that found Oxford House residents have greater improvements in self-regulation compared to individuals receiving regular aftercare (Jason et al., 2006). These benefits are enhanced by staying in an Oxford House for 6 months or longer (Jason, Olson, et al., 2007), suggesting that residents might improve their ability to inhibit their aggressive impulses over time. Such recovery outcomes might be a result of the unique contingencies that are utilized within Oxford Houses as methods of self-governance (Ferrari et al., 2004; Jason, Olson, Ferrari, Layne, Davis, & Alvarez, 2003). Living in mutually supportive settings that encourage prosocial behavior among abstinent support networks (Majer, Jason, Ferrari, Venable, & Olson, 2002) and increase self-efficacy and personal responsibility (Davis & Jason, 2005; Ferrari, Jason, Olson, Davis, & Alvarez, 2002) might improve interpersonal relationships. Residents may become more prosocial in their behavior over time and expand their ability to take the perspectives of others (Olson et al., 2005).

Perhaps one of the most direct mechanisms by which both criminal and aggressive behaviors can be reduced among individuals in recovery is through continued abstinence, as previous findings suggest (e.g., BJS, 1998). Because approximately 80% of the full sample reported total abstinence from substance use throughout the course of the study (Jason, Davis, et al., 2007), it is not surprising that there were low levels of aggressive and criminal behaviors at the one-year follow-up. It is possible that continued sobriety by itself may have prevented some of these problematic behaviors from occurring within our sample.

Several limitations in this study warrant consideration. First, it is possible that some sample selection bias existed because this was a convenience sample. Furthermore, the research design used in the present study did not include a control group for comparative purposes or collect non-self-report collateral or biological verification of substance abstinence. Moreover, attrition is always problematic regarding the interpretation of results in longitudinal research due to inherent biases. However, at baseline, the group that later dropped out did not differ from the group that completed the study on a number of different variables. While this does not resolve the attrition issue, it appears that there were no major differences between the groups.

In summary, results of the present study suggest that spending more time in a supportive setting like an Oxford House might help to reduce the incidence of criminal and aggressive behaviors among individuals in recovery. These findings may be the result of some of the tangible benefits provided by an Oxford House environment (e.g., low-crime neighborhoods, higher income), improved self-regulation and prosocial behavior resulting from self-governing networks of abstinent peers, or even simply the maintenance of abstinence. Future research should evaluate these mechanisms more closely, with the goal of understanding specific pathways by which mutually supportive recovery environments like Oxford Houses could be beneficial for different populations of individuals in recovery for addiction.

REFERENCES

Bleiberg, J. L., Devlin, P., Croan, J., & Briscoe, R. (1994). Relationship between treatment length and outcome in a therapeutic community. *International Journal of Addictions, 29,* 729–740.

Bureau of Justice Statistics. (1998). *Alcohol and crime: An analysis of national data on the prevalence of alcohol involvement in crime* (NCJ 168632). Washington, DC: Author.

Bureau of Justice Statistics. (2005). *Substance dependence, abuse, and treatment of jail inmates, 2002* (NCJ 209588). Washington, DC: Author.

Bushman, B., & Cooper, H. (1990). Effects of alcohol on human aggression: An integrative research review. *Psychological Bulletin, 10,* 341–354.

Davis, M. I., & Jason, L. A. (2005). Sex differences in social support and self-efficacy within a recovery community. *American Journal of Community Psychology, 36,* 259–274.

Eklund, J. M., & Klinteberg, B. (2005). Personality characteristics as risk indications of alcohol use and violent behavior in male and female adolescents. *Journal of Individual Differences, 26,* 63–73.

Ferrari, J. R., Jason, L. A., Blake, R., Davis, M. I., & Olson, B. D. (2006). "This is my neighborhood"; Comparing United States and Australian Oxford House neighborhoods. *Journal of Prevention and Intervention in the Community, 31,* 41–49.

Ferrari, J. R., Jason, L. A., Davis, M. I., Olson, B. D., & Alvarez, J. (2004). Similarities and differences in governance among residents in drug and/or alcohol misuse: Self vs. staff rules and regulations. *Therapeutic Communities: The International Journal for Therapeutic and Supportive Organizations, 25,* 179–192.

Ferrari, J. R., Jason, L. A., Olson, B. D., Davis, M. I., & Alvarez, J. (2002). Sense of community among Oxford House residents recovering from substance abuse: Making a house a home. In A. T. Fischer, C. C. Sonn, & B. J. Bishop (Eds.), *Psychological Sense of Community* (pp. 109–122). New York: Kluwer/Plenum.

Hubbard, R. L., Craddock, S. G., Flynn, P. M., Anderson, J., & Etheridge, R. M. (1997). Overview of 1-year follow-up outcomes in the Drug Abuse Treatment Outcome Study (DATOS). *Psychology of Addictive Behaviors, 11*, 261–278.

Inciardi, J., McBride, D., McCoy, H. V., & Chitwood, D. (1994). Recent research on the crack/cocaine/crime connection. *Studies on Crime and Crime Prevention, 3*, 63–82.

Jason, L. A., Davis, M. I., Ferrari, J. R., & Anderson, E. (2007). The need for substance abuse after-care: A longitudinal analysis of Oxford House. *Addictive Behaviors, 32*, 803–818.

Jason, L. A., Davis, M. I., Ferrari, J. R., & Bishop, P. D. (2001). Oxford House: A review of research and implications for substance abuse recovery and community research. *Journal of Drug Education, 31*, 1–27.

Jason, L. A., Ferrari, J. R., Smith, B., Marsh, P., Dvorchak, P. A., Groessl, E. J., et al. (1997). An exploratory study of male recovering substance abusers living in a self-help, self-governed setting. *Journal of Mental Health Administration, 24*, 332–339.

Jason, L. A., Olson, B. D., Ferrari, J. R., Layne, A., Davis, M. I., & Alvarez, J. (2003). A case-study of self-governance in a drug abuse recovery home. *North American Journal of Psychology, 5*, 499–514.

Jason, L. A., Olson, B. D., Ferrari, J. R., & Lo Sasso, A. T. (2006). Communal housing settings enhance substance abuse recovery. *American Journal of Public Health, 96*, 1727–1729.

Jason, L. A., Olson, B. D., Ferrari, J. R., Majer, J. M., Alvarez, J., & Stout, J. (2007). An examination of main and interactive effects of substance abuse recovery. *Addiction, 102*, 1114–1121.

Kaplan, H. (1995). Contemporary themes and emerging directions in longitudinal research on deviant behavior. In H. Kaplan (Ed.), *Drugs, crime, and other deviant adaptations: Longitudinal research* (pp. 233–241). New York: Plenum.

Majer, J. M., Jason, L. A., Ferrari, J. R., Venable, L. B., & Olson, B. D. (2002). Social support and self-efficacy for abstinence: Is peer identification an issue? *Journal of Substance Abuse Treatment, 23*, 209–215.

McLellan, A. T., Kushner, H., Metzger, D., Peters, R., Smith, I., Grissom, G., et al. (1992). The fifth edition of the Addiction Severity Index. *Journal of Substance Abuse Treatment, 9*, 199–213.

Miller, W. R. (1996). *Form 90: A structured assessment interview for drinking and related behaviors, test manual* (NIH Publication No. 96-4004). Bethesda, MD: NIAAA.

Miller, W. R., & Del Boca, F. K. (1994). Measurement of drinking behavior using the Form 90 family of instruments. *Journal of Studies on Alcohol Supplement, 12*, 112–118.

Miller, M., & Potter-Efron, R. (1989). Aggression and violence associated with substance abuse. *Journal of Chemical Dependency Treatment, 3*, 1–36.

Murphy, C., Winters, J., O'Farrell, T., Fals-Stewart, W., & Murphy, M. (2005). Alcohol consumption and intimate partner violence by alcoholic men: Comparing violent and non-violent conflicts. *Psychology of Addictive Behaviors, 19*, 35–42.

Olson, B. D., Jason, L. A., Ferrari, J. R., & Hutcheson, T. D. (2005). Bridging professional and mutual-help: An application of the transtheoretical model to the mutual-help organization. *Applied and Preventative Psychology, 11*, 167–178.

Oxford House, Inc. (2006). *Oxford House manual.* Silver Spring, MD: Oxford House, Inc.

Putt, C. A., Dowd, E. T., & McCormick, R. A. (2001). Impact of pre-existing levels of hostility and aggression on substance abuse treatment outcome. *Counselling Psychology Quarterly, 14*(2), 139–147.

Thomson, L. (1999). Substance abuse and criminality. *Current Opinion in Psychiatry, 12*, 653–657.

Titus, J. C., & Dennis, M. L. (2000). *Global appraisal of individual needs quick screen (GAIN-QS): Instructions for version 1.* Bloomington, IL: Chestnut Health Systems.

Weinfurt, K. P. (2000). Repeated measures analyses: ANOVA, MANOVA, and HLM. In L. Grimm & P. Yarnold (Eds.), *Reading and understanding more multivariate statistics* (pp. 317–361). Washington, DC: American Psychological Association.

The Relationship of Gender and Ethnicity to Employment Among Adults Residing in Communal-Living Recovery Homes

OLYA BELYAEV-GLANTSMAN, MA, LEONARD A. JASON, PhD,
and JOSEPH R. FERRARI, PhD

DePaul University

This study examined employment and sources of income for different genders and ethnic groups residing in a substance abuse recovery homes called Oxford Houses. Men compared to women reported significantly higher mean income from employment as well as total income. African Americans compared to European Americans reported significantly more work in the past 30 days; however, the rate of pay between these two ethnic groups was not significantly different. Longer length of stay in Oxford House was related to higher incomes. Implications of these findings are discussed.

It is estimated that over 22.5 million Americans ages 12 or older (approximately 9.4% of the population) are classified with substance dependence or abuse. These maladaptive patterns of substance use lead to clinically significant impairment (National Survey on Drug Use and Health [NSDUH], 2004) and may interfere with a person's ability to work (Zlotnik, Robertson, & Tam, 2002). Bray, Zarkin, Dennis, and French (2000) found that for both men and women substance use with symptoms of dependence was associated with lower employment rates and represented a barrier to leaving welfare. Finally, individuals who abused drugs and were employed cost their

Portions of this article reflected the masters thesis of the first author under the supervision of the second and third authors. The authors appreciate financial support from the National Institute on Drug Abuse (grant number DA13231).

employers about twice as much in medical and worker compensation claims as their drug-free coworkers (NIDA, 2004).

Employment is among the most important factors associated with alcohol and substance abuse addictions (Brady & Mathews, 2002). For instance, employment rates for those adults addicted to substances were lower than for those adults not addicted (NSDUH, 2003). The National Survey on Drug Use and Health revealed that in 2004 an estimated 19.2% of unemployed adults were substance users, whereas 8.0% of full-time and 10.3% of part-time employed adults were classified with dependence or abuse.

Furthermore, employment seems to be related to successful recovery. Sterling, Gottheil, Glassman, Weinstein, Serota, and Lundy (2001) found that employed adults were doing significantly better in their recovery process than unemployed adults. In addition, the loss of employment was associated with relapse (Fisher & Anglin, 1987). Thus, attainment and sustainability of steady employment may serve as a central mediator of positive substance use outcome (Gregoire & Snively, 2001; Platt, 1995; Sterling et al., 2001). While steady employment may facilitate and help sustain abstinence, recovering individuals may encounter multiple barriers, particularly in regards to gaining and retaining employment. Obstacles such as lack of job-searching skills, scarcity of low-level jobs, prejudice against the person in recovery, employer's fear of applicant's relapse, and lack of social support may prevent a person in recovery from successfully gaining employment.

The Oxford House model for recovery seems to provide a mixture of residential therapeutic community and 12-step approaches (Oxford House, 2004). It is built on a democratic framework, with over 1,200 rented dwellings located across the USA (Jason, Ferrari, Davis, & Olson, 2006). No professional staff lives within any residence, and house decisions are based on traditions specified in the house rules and are voted on by house members. Largely because of its self-run nature, the program is far less costly to initiate and run compared to the operational costs of the staffed therapeutic community model (Oxford House, 2004). Three rules of the house are that members must (a) abstain from drinking or using drugs, (b) avoid disruptive behavior, and (c) pay rent through their own employment or social service benefits (Ferrari, Jason, Davis, Olson, & Alvarez, 2004).

It may be important to examine self-run recovery homes such as Oxford House because living in such settings may help with a number of barriers toward gaining and maintaining stable employment faced by individuals in recovery. Because there is a need to pay rent for residency in an Oxford House, there is an incentive to find a steady source of income. It may also be easier to find a better job while residing in an Oxford House, particularly because the employer may be assured that the person has a stable and substance-free living arrangement. The residents of the house may also serve as a resource by helping new residents find and sustain employment through recommendations and referrals. Oxford House may work as a platform for persons recovering from abuse as well as an aid in gaining and retaining employment. At the same time, Oxford House creates an option for persons in recovery to stay abstinent in a substance-free environment among similar others while they are becoming self-efficient and productive members of society. Finally, based on previous studies, living in an abstinent setting, away from high-risk environments, may facilitate addiction recovery (see Ferrari, Jason, Olson, Davis, & Alvarez, 2002; Jason, Davis, Ferrari, & Bishop 2001).

The present study explored effects of gender, ethnicity, and length of stay on the number of days worked in the past 30 and the sources of income among Oxford House members. It was predicted that men compared to women would report more days worked and higher income, especially from employment, and lower income from other sources such as unemployment compensation, pension, the Department of Public Aid (DPA), or family, friends, and partner. It also was predicted that European Americans compared to African Americans would report more days worked and higher income, especially from employment, and lower income from other sources such as unemployment compensation, pension, DPA, or family, friends, and partner. Finally, it was predicted that those adults who stayed in Oxford House for 6 months or longer would report more days worked and higher income, especially from employment, and lower income from other sources such as unemployment compensation, pension, DPA, or family, friends, and partner, than adults who stayed in Oxford House for less than 6 months.

METHOD

Participants

This study was a part of a larger National Institute on Drug Abuse (NIDA)–funded national study of Oxford Houses (see Jason, Davis, Ferrari, & Anderson, 2007 for details) from 2001 to 2006. There were 897 participants involved in the study (604 males, 293 females), with a mean age of 38.4 years old. Participants were recruited from five cluster areas across the United States: Washington and Oregon, Texas, Illinois, Pennsylvania and New Jersey, and North Carolina. These clusters indicated locations of the majority of Oxford Houses across the USA. On average, participants spent 10.85 months ($SD = 15.04$) residing in an Oxford House.

The present sample was ethnically diverse, with 58.4% being European American, 34.0% African American, 3.5% Latino, and 4% other. Marital status of the sample included 49% single/never married, 46.2% divorced or widowed or separated, and 4.8% married. The average education level reported by participants was 12.6 years. With respect to employment, 69.3% reported being employed full-time, 13.9% employed part-time, 11.6% unemployed, and 3.8% retired or disabled at the time of the survey. The average monthly income across participants was $981.80.

Based on the preliminary review of the data, the majority of the present sample was diagnosed with alcohol and drug abuse or dependence, as well as significant histories of co-morbid mental health and behavioral problems. This sample reflected the overall sociodemographic makeup and substance use disorders of individuals from the national sample of Oxford House residents from which the sample was drawn.

Materials

Participants completed the Addiction Severity Index—Lite (ASI; McLellan, Kushner, Metzger, Peters, Smith, Grissom, et al., 1992), a semi-structured interview protocol widely used throughout the United States and other countries to assess a number of substance-abuse related behaviors. It is an intake assessment instrument used to develop a treatment plan and is designed to obtain information about lifetime problem behaviors as well as those in the past 30 days prior to assessment. The survey covered several areas of a person's life, namely, their medical history, their employment or financial support, their drug and alcohol use, their legal issues, matters related to their family or social domain, and their psychiatric issues. The ASI has often been used in substance abuse related studies and has been shown to have excellent test–retest reliability of (0.83) or higher with the coefficient alpha $\geq$ 0.80 (McLellan et al., 1992). Sample questions included "How long was your longest full-time job?" and "How many days were you paid for working in the past 30 days?"

Sociodemographic and other pertinent information were gathered via specific portions of the ASI fifth Edition. Because of the nature of this study, the employment section of the ASI scale was a major focus. For the present study, demographic and background information from the ASI included, age, sex, ethnicity, months of education or technical education completed, distribution of financial support, pay rates, and length of residence.

RESULTS

A $2 \times 2 \times 2$ (gender by ethnicity by length of stay) analysis of covariance (ANCOVA) was conducted for each of the 6 dependent measures (i.e., income from employment and total income, number of days paid for work, income from unemployment compensation, income from DPA, and income from partner, family, and friends). Because of the possible confounding differences due to age or education level, analyses controlled for these variables.

TABLE 1 Financial Characteristics of the OH Residents

	Gender		Ethnicity	
	Female	Male	White	Black
Education (months)	148.61	153.77*	153.95*	148.74
Days paid for work (number of days)	15.80	16.56	15.64	17.54*
Money from ($)				
employment	615.74	941.56**	820.10	869.99
unemployment compensation	23.2	47.23	40.8	29.63
DPA	10.96	8.34	9.68	9.62
pension, benefits or social security	97.57	72.32	106.97	62.918
partner, family or friends	70.18	45.2	66.06	49.31
Total monthly income ($)	814.8	1120.95**	943.16	992.58

Note: $*p < .05. **p < .001.$

Table 1 presents findings regarding gender and ethnic differences in education and financial variables. Males reported significantly more months of formal education completed compared to females [$M = 153.77$, $SD = 23.95$ versus $M = 148.61$, $SD = 27.59$ months, $F(1,804) = 6.97$, $p < .05$] European Americans reported significantly more months of formal education completed compared to African Americans [$M = 153.95$, $SD = 23.08$ versus $M = 148.74$, $SD = 27.01$ months, $F(1,804) = 7.07$, $p < .005$]. There was no significant difference in the number of days worked between the two genders. There was, however, a significant difference in the number of days worked between the two ethnic groups with African Americans reporting higher number of days paid for work [$M = 17.76$, $SE = .75$ versus $M = 15.32$, $SE = .56$ days, $F(1,732) = 6.6$, $p < .01$, partial $\eta^2 = .009$]. There was a significant difference in the amount of money from employment and the total amount of income between the two genders with men reporting higher amounts compared to women [$M = \$948.01$, $SE = 47.32$ versus $M = \$646.42$, $SE = 69.15$, $F(1,732) = 12.80$, $p < .001$, partial $\eta^2 = .945$ and $M = \$1123.50$, $SE = 40.03$ versus $M = \$811.33$, $SE = 58.50$, $F(1,732) = 19.17$, $p < .001$, partial $\eta^2 = .026$].

Table 2 indicates that the number of days paid for work increased significantly for those who stayed in OH for 6 months or more compared to those who stayed in OH for less than 6 months [$M = 18.42$, $SE = .58$ versus $M = 14.20$, $SE = .59$, $F(1,729), = 25.57$, $p < .001$, partial $\eta^2 = .034$]. At the same time, those who stayed in OH for 6 months or longer reported significantly higher amounts of both income from employment and overall income compared to those who stayed in OH for less than 6 months [$M = \$1,035.27$, $SE = 52.35$ versus $M = \$635.13$, $SE = 53.46$, $F(1,729) = 27.81$, partial $\eta^2 = .037$, $p < .001$ and $M = \$1,171.42$, $SE = 44.74$ versus $M = \$861.77$, $SE = 45.69$, $F(1,729) = 22.80$, $p < .001$, partial $\eta^2 = .30$ respectively].

TABLE 2 Lengths of Stay in OH

	Length of stay	
	<6 months	>=6 months
Days paid for work (number of days)	14.20	18.42**
Money from ($)		
employment	635.13	1,035.27**
unemployment compensation	55.00	28.09
DPA	6.70	12.78
pension, benefits or social security	87.00	88.95
partner, family or friends	73.92	38.56
Total monthly income ($)	861.77	1171.42**

Note: **p < .001.

DISCUSSION

The current study suggested that Oxford House may help provide a setting that increases economic opportunities for residents, as financial character-istics improved with length of stay. Adults who continued residence for 6 months or more reported a higher number of days working, higher in-come from employment, and higher overall income, compared to adults who stayed in OH for less than 6 months. Apparently, with longer time since entering a recovery setting such as Oxford House, income and number of days worked per month improve.

In terms of months of education, income from employment, and the to-tal income, men did significantly better than women. Both men and women, however, did not significantly differ on number of days paid for work, in-come from unemployment compensation, income from DPA, and income from partner, family, and friends. Perhaps a gender pay gap existed, as re-ported in U.S. society, such that men earn significantly more money for the same amount of work than women (Lips, 2003). According to Bem (2005), organized society is a better fit for men, automatically placing women at certain disadvantages, including financial obstacles such as income. Based on the present study, these disadvantages were mirrored in substance abuse recovery populations in the United States. Women compared to men might be disadvantaged at the beginning of the recovery process and might require additional assistance, particularly in gaining financial independence.

European Americans also reported a significantly higher mean number of months of formal education compared to African Americans. There was no significant difference, however, between these two ethnic groups in regards to income from employment. Furthermore, African Americans reported working significantly longer on average than European Americans. Thus, while African American's employment rates were significantly higher, their income from employment was not—suggesting that African Americans were getting paid less for the same amount of work as their European American counterparts.

An explanation for this outcome may be that a gap favoring the latter group exists between African Americans and European Americans on financial characteristics such as the employment-to-population ratio, the unemployment-to-population ratio, and income, among others (Current Population Survey [CPS], 2007). According to the U.S. Bureau of Labor Statistics (2007), in 2000 African Americans earned 71.6 percent of what European Americans earned. This trend can still be seen in current years, as based on the CPS, in 2006, median weekly earnings of European Americans were $690, while median weekly earning of African Americans were $554 (CPS, 2007).

LIMITATIONS AND FUTURE DIRECTIONS

Of course, there are several limitations in the present study. For instance, despite the seeming overall ethnic diversity of the sample (i.e., 58.5% being European American, 34.1% African American, 3.5% Latino, 2% American Indian, and 2% other), only the two largest groups (i.e., European Americans and African Americans) were included in the analyses due to the small sample size of the other subgroups. The authors chose not to collapse the minority subgroups into an "other" category, as such would have not provided enough information regarding each of the separate ethnic groups. Inclusion of other ethnic subgroups within the recovery population is necessary for gaining a better understanding of ethnic difference in regard to financial status. Oversampling certain ethnic groups might be of benefit to future research.

Despite the limitations, our prospective analysis suggested that programs like Oxford House may provide not only an abstinent environment that promotes recovery from substance abuse but also work as a stepping stone toward a more stable financial status among adults in recovery. Despite overall improvement on a number of financial characteristics, certain subgroups (e.g., African Americans) may have greater or lesser economic obstacles to overcome. Future research might identify specific barriers toward financial independence subgroups may face. Furthermore, qualitative data may provide even greater insight into the potential barriers and resilience factors in overcoming such barriers toward financial independence among the recovering population.

REFERENCES

Bem, S. L. (1994). In a male-centered world, female differences are transformed into female disadvantages. In P. S. Rothenberg (Ed.), *Race, class, and gender in the United States: An integrated study* (pp. 60–63) New York: St. Martin's Press.

Brady, S. S., & Mathews, K. A. (2002). The influence of socioeconomic status and ethnicity on adolescents' exposure to stressful life events. *Journal of Pediatric Psychology*, *27*, 575–583.

Bray, J. W., Zarkin, G. A., Dennis, M. L., & French, M. T. (2000). Symptoms of dependence, multiple substance use, and labor market outcomes. *American Journal of Drug & Alcohol Abuse*, *26*, 77–95.

Ferrari, J. R., Jason, L. A., Davis, M. I., Olson, B. D., & Alvarez, J. (2004). Similarities and differences in governance among residents in drug and/or alcohol misuse: Self vs. staff rules and regulations. *Therapeutic Communities: The International Journal for Therapeutic and Supportive Organizations*, *25*, 179–192.

Ferrari, J. R., Jason, L. A., Olson, B. D., Davis, M. I., & Alvarez, J. (2002). Sense of community among Oxford House residents recovering from substance abuse: Making a house a home. In A. T. Fisher, C. C. Sonn, & B. J. Bishop (Eds.), *Psychological sense of community: Research, applications, and implications* (pp. 109–122). New York: Kluwer Academic/Plenum Publishers.

Fisher, D. G., & Anglin, M. D. (1987). Parental influences on substance use: Gender differences and stage theory. *Journal of Drug Education*, *22*, 69–86.

Gregoire, T. K., & Snively, C. A. (2001). The relationship of social support and economic self-sufficiency to substance abuse outcomes in a long-term recovery program for women. *Journal of Drug Education*, *31*, 221–237.

Jason, L. A., Davis, M. I., Ferrari, J. R., & Anderson, E. (2007). The need for substance abuse after-care: A longitudinal analysis of Oxford House. *Addictive Behaviors*, *32*, 803–818.

Jason, L. A., Davis, M. I., Ferrari, J. R., & Bishop, P. D. (2001). Oxford House: A review of research and implications for substance abuse recovery and community research. *Journal of Drug Education*, *31*, 1–27.

Jason, L. A., Ferrari, J. R., Davis, M. I., & Olson, B. D. (2006). Communal housing settings enhance substance abuse recovery. *Journal of Prevention & Intervention in the Community*, *31*, xix–xx.

Lips, H. M. (2003). The gender pay gap: Concrete indicator of women's progress toward equality. *Analyses of Social Issues and Public Policy*, *3*, 87–109.

McLellan, A. T., Kushner, H., Metzger, D., Peters, R., Smith, I., Grissom, G., et al (1992). The fifth edition of the Addiction Severity Index. *Journal of Substance Abuse Treatment*, *9*, 199–213.

National Survey on Drug Use and Health. (2004). Retrieved February 15, 2006, from http://oas.samhsa.gov

Oxford House. (2004). Retrieved October 2, 2004, from http://www.oxfordhouse.org/userfiles/file/purpose_and_structure.php structure

Platt, J. (1995). Vocational rehabilitation of drug abusers. *Psychological Bulletin*, *117*, 416–433.

Rogler, L. H., Cortes, D. E., & Malgady, R. G. (1991). Acculturation and mental health status among Hispanics: Convergence and new direction of research. *American Psychologist*, *46*, 585–597.

Sterling, R. C., Gottheil, E., Glassman, S. D., Weinstein, S. P., Serota, R. D., & Lundy, A. (2001). Correlates of employment: A cohort study. *American Journal of Drug Abuse*, *27*, 137–146.

Workplace Trends. (2004). Retrieved October, 2004, from http://www.nida.nih.gov/Infofax/workplace.html

The Neighborhood Environments
of Mutual-Help Recovery Houses: Comparisons
by Perceived Socioeconomic Status

JOSEPH R. FERRARI, PhD, DAVID R. GROH, PhD, and
LEONARD A. JASON, PhD

DePaul University

This study examined the setting and house-level characteristics of 160 self-governed, mutual-support substance abuse recovery homes, called Oxford Houses (OHs), across the United States. These dwellings were located in four different neighborhood types: upper or middle class (n = 23 houses), urban working or lower class (n = 71 houses), suburban upper or middle-class (n = 39 Houses), and suburban working or lower class (n = 27 houses). Interior dwelling characteristics and amenities located within a 2-block radius were similar across the four neighborhood types. However, houses in urban, working, and lower class neighborhoods reported more alcohol- or drug-intoxicated persons. Most importantly, despite the greater potential for environmental temptations and easier access for substances, none of the neighborhood factors including neighborhood socioeconomic status significantly predicted relapse rates over a 12-month period.

Oxford House (OH) is a residential, community-based option for individuals dealing with substance abuse problems (see Ferrari, Jason, Davis, Olson, &

Funding for this manuscript was made possible in part by NIH grant awards from the National Institute on Drug Abuse (NIDA # DA13231). The authors express much gratitude to Ed Anderson for data analysis, to Brad Olson, Meg Davis, John Majer, and Josefina Alvarez for feedback on conceptualizations, and to the Oxford House members who allowed information on their homes for inclusion in this study.

Alvarez, 2004; Jason, Ferrari, Davis, & Olson, 2006). A low cost, self-run, democratic recovery home model, OH has grown since 1975 to over 1,250 homes across the USA, Canada, and Australia. Regarding the operation and maintenance of OHs, no professional staff is involved, enabling residents to create their own rules for communal governance. Residents live together in a democratic, single-sex home and provide each other with a supportive abstinent mutual-support network. The residents may stay indefinitely, provided that they pay rent, abstain from alcohol and drug use, and avoid disruptive behavior (Ferrari et al.). Failure to comply with these guidelines is grounds for expulsion from the OH. Residents continually support each other to find and maintain employment, as members rely on this income source to pay rent.

Ferrari and colleagues focused on setting or house-level variables within OHs. Ferrari, Jason, Sasser, Davis, and Olson (2006) found many similarities within the physical structures and interior or exterior designs of U.S. OHs. These house characteristics and amenities created a sense of home not often found in traditional treatments centers. Ferrari et al. (2004) found that both Illinois OHs and therapeutic communities prohibited self-injurious behaviors (e.g., physical self-harm or overmedication of drugs) and destructive acts (e.g., destroying site property or others' possessions). OHs, however, more typically permitted residents greater personal freedoms.

The Oxford House national organization dictated that new houses be established in safe, low-crime, economically stable neighborhoods with minimal opportunities for relapse (Oxford House, 1988). Ferrari, Jason, Blake, Davis, and Olson (2006) found that regardless of geographic location, U.S. and Australian OHs were situated in communities that had access to public amenities (e.g., grocery stores, hospitals, and restaurants) and little illegal drug and crime activity. Local communities reported that OH residents blended well into the neighborhood and made good neighbors (Jason, Roberts, & Olson, 2005). The majority of OH neighbors interviewed gained resources, friendships, or a greater sense of security following contact with the OH residents. No evidence of property devaluation was found for neighborhoods including OHs. In fact, those who knew of the OH saw an increase in property value over an average of 3 years.

Research has fairly thoroughly examined the relationship between OHs and the surrounding community. None of the studies cited above, however, explored how the socioeconomic status of the surrounding community specifically affected the outcomes of these residential settings. Studies indicate that lower neighborhood socioeconomic status is negatively related to individual mental health and perceived health (Drukker & van Os, 2003). More specifically, living in a lower socioeconomic neighborhood was linked to heart disease, diabetes, obesity (Brown, Guy, & Broad, 2005), smoking (Brown et al.; Chuang, Cubbin, Ahn, & Winkleby, 2005; Shohaimi, Luben, Wareham, Day, Bingham, Welch, et al., 2003), alcohol or drug problems (Brown et al.; Smart, Adlaf, & Walsh, 1995), risky sexual behaviors (Baumer & South, 2001), and less access to exercise resources and facilities (Estabrooks, Lee, & Gyurcsik, 2003). Thus, this article focused on how neighborhood characteristics such as socioeconomic status impacted abstinence outcomes for residents of OHs. In addition, no previous study examined how environmental temptations (e.g., neighborhoods with easy access to drugs or the presence of intoxicated persons on the streets) influenced the probability of abstinence among these residents. The present study explored these environmental issues within a U.S. nationwide sample of OHs that differed on the socioeconomic characteristics of their neighborhoods. In addition, the long-term sobriety rates of these OHs were examined over a 12-month period.

METHOD

Oxford Houses in the Present Study

Data for the present study were from a 16-month NIDA-funded community evaluation of residents living in one of 213 U.S. OHs (see Jason, Davis, Ferrari, & Anderson, 2007, for details). We only included the 160 OHs for which we had environmental and substance use data from the majority of house residents, representing 75.1% of OHs in the original sample of 213. Previous studies indicated that independent judges reliably categorized and assessed setting characteristics (see Ferrari, Jason, Blake, et al., 2006; Ferrari, Jason, Sasser, et al., 2006). Based on responses from OH representatives on an environmental audit, we grouped the current sample by socioeconomic status in this manner: 23 OHs (18 men's homes, 5 women's homes) located in an urban and upper- or middle-class neighborhood, 71 urban and working- or lower-class OHs (47 men's homes, 24 women's homes), 39 suburban and upper- or middle-class OHs (27 men's homes, 12 women's homes), and 27 suburban and working- or lower-class OHs (20 men's homes, 7 women's homes).

Preliminary chi square analysis indicated that the four socioeconomic groups did not significantly differ by gender. The present sample reflected 70.0% men and 30.0% women facilities, a ratio consistent with other U.S. Oxford House samples (see Jason, Ferrari, et al., 2006). A MANOVA on several descriptive variables indicated no significant difference among these four groups regarding the number of years the setting was in operation, geographic region, the number of adult or child residents within an OH, or the type of substances abused (i.e., alcohol, drug, poly-substance). These dwellings operated as an OH an average of 7.06 years ($SD = 3.77$) and were located in a variety of U.S. geographic locations. Furthermore, these OH dwellings included an average of 7.12 adults ($SD = 1.95$) with few if any children ($M = 0.13$, $SD = 0.57$). Adult residents identified as former alcohol ($M = 14.8\%$, $SD = 19.1$) or drug users ($M = 32.7\%$; $SD = 32.7$), but mostly poly-substance users ($M = 58.2\%$, $SD = 36.8$).

Environmental Audit

The survey used in the present study was a brief version of a reliable instrument developed and utilized by Ferrari and colleagues (Ferrari et al., 2004; Ferrari, Jason, Blake, et al., 2006; Ferrari, Jason, Sasser, et al., 2006b) for use with group recovery dwellings. This environmental audit requested responses to forced-choice and frequency items in a number of domains, including demographic–static information about the house members, such as the percentage of residents in recovery from alcohol, drugs, and poly-substances, plus the number of inhabitants within an OH. Sections of this audit gathered information on the interior and immediate exterior OH characteristics. Respondents walked through the home and recorded the number of certain features commonly found in homes (e.g., bedrooms, kitchen, yard). The next section focused on the amenities found within the immediate two-block radius of the OH (see Ferrari, Jason, Sasser, et al., 2006). Respondents were asked if they would encounter various amenities in their neighborhood (e.g., police station, hospital, mall) if they "walked around the block." Finally, respondents reported on the characteristics of the surrounding neighborhood (e.g., empty buildings, clean streets, drug dealers on the streets).

Cumulative Abstinence Rates of Oxford Houses

We also assessed the cumulative abstinence rates of the men and women in this U.S. national Oxford House sample. Individuals were tracked over a 12-month period; some persons stayed in an OH while others moved out (either by their own means or due to eviction for violating house rules or relapsing). For each OH in the study, we computed the mean cumulative abstinence rate for either alcohol and drug use across four measurement waves at 4-month intervals (see Jason et al., 2007). Controlling for initial time spent in OH, we measured the average rate of change in cumulative abstinence for each house, represented by latent slope variables. Slopes closer to 1.00 indicated longer lengths of sobriety (i.e., less use or relapse) for OH members over one year. Jason et al. effectively calculated abstinence rates for individuals in recovery, and we altered this process to assess setting or house-level abstinence. The average slopes for house-level alcohol and drug abstinence were significantly related ($r = 0.89$, $p < .001$), and we combined abstinence from alcohol and drugs together into one variable.

Procedure

The environmental audits were mailed to the OH presidents of all 213 OHs. No identifiable information about any individual OH resident was requested, and confidentially was maintained for all data. Most surveys were completed and returned by postage-paid mail from the house president (60.2%) or another house officer (31.6%; e.g., secretary or treasurer) with a small package of coffee subsequently sent for house participation. Pilot testing indicated that it took less than 20 minutes to complete and mail the survey, which was collected over a 4-month period. An ANOVA analysis was conducted to test whether OHs in the four neighborhood types differed with respect to 12-month house-level cumulative abstinence rates. In addition, a linear regression analysis tested whether the presence of the reported environmental variables (i.e., immediate neighborhood amenities and community factors) predicted 12-month house-level cumulative abstinence rates.

RESULTS

We initially conducted preliminary analyses (chi square and ANOVA: p levels set at 0.01 to control for Type 1 error) comparing the 160 OHs included in the present study with the 51 OHs omitted from the study on setting variables. No significant differences were obtained regarding gender of the residents, proportion of residents in recovery from alcohol versus drug use, length of time the setting operated as an OH, geographic region of the home, or economic status of the neighborhood. Moreover, there was no significant difference between the included and excluded OHs regarding average rates of cumulative abstinence from alcohol and drugs within the settings.

Immediate Amenities and Community Characteristics

Tables 1 and 2 present the mean percentage of OHs in each socioeconomic group reporting the presence of observed immediate amenities and community conditions. Chi-square analyses indicated no significant differences across the four classes on immediate amenities and observed neighborhood characteristics. However, significant differences existed between the four classes regarding the presence of intoxicated persons, χ^2 (3, $n = 157$) = 20.57, $p < .001$, "drugged" persons, χ^2 (3, $n = 158$) = 21.47, $p < .001$, and empty building lots on the streets, χ^2 (3, $n = 157$) = 11.25, $p = .01$. OHs in urban working or lower class areas most frequently reported their presence.

Neighborhood Factors and Cumulative Abstinence

The mean cumulative abstinence slope for the OHs was 0.91 ($SD = 0.11$), which approached total abstinence (a value of 1.00) over the 12-month timeframe. This low rate of use may not be surprising, given that any substance use led to expulsion from Oxford House. However, while most OHs

TABLE 1 Mean Percentage of Oxford Houses Reporting Immediate Access to Amenities by Neighborhood Socioeconomic Status

	Urban		Suburban	
	Upper or middle (n = 23)	Working or lower (n = 71)	Upper or middle (n = 39)	Working or lower (n = 27)
Police station	4.5	15.9	33.3	24.0
Medical clinic	36.4	24.6	23.1	24.0
Hospital	27.3	20.3	10.3	16.0
Social Welfare Dept.	9.1	10.1	2.6	12.0
Homeless shelter	0.0	11.6	0.0	4.0
Homeless food service	9.1	10.1	2.6	8.0
Well lit streets, at night	100.0	95.8	94.9	85.2
Public parking	95.7	95.8	94.9	100.0
Public transportation	95.7	98.6	87.2	81.5
Gas or service station	50.0	69.6	71.8	60.0
Library	13.6	27.6	30.8	24.0
Large supermarket	45.5	37.7	48.7	40.0
Large shopping mall	18.2	7.3	20.5	16.0
Mini-market or strip mall	54.5	68.1	56.4	40.0

TABLE 2 Mean Percentage of Oxford Houses Reporting Community Conditions by Neighborhood Socioeconomic Status

	Urban		Suburban	
	Upper or middle (n = 23)	Working or lower (n = 71)	Upper or middle (n = 39)	Working or lower (n = 27)
Economically depressed feeling	8.7	15.7	0.0	14.8
Empty buildings or lots*	8.7	18.8	0.0	3.7
Streets deserted during the day	21.7	31.4	31.6	25.9
Streets deserted during the night	34.8	38.6	52.6	29.6
Other buildings are well kept	91.3	87.1	100.0	92.6
Streets clean or free of litter	91.3	80.3	100.0	85.2
Trees or greenery planted on streets	91.3	88.4	92.1	92.6
Homeless persons observed sleeping in the neighborhood at night	8.7	8.8	0.0	3.7
Homeless persons seen "hanging-out" on streets during the day	13.0	14.5	0.0	3.7
Pawn shops visible	17.4	25.3	5.3	18.5
Intoxicated persons observed on streets**	17.4	37.7	2.6	11.1
Drug persons observed on streets**	17.4	40.0	2.6	14.8
Drug dealing observed on streets	13.0	27.1	5.3	11.5

*$p < .01$; **$p < .001$.

TABLE 3 Summary of Linear Regression Analysis for Neighborhood Variables Predicting Cumulative Abstinence

Neighborhood variable	B	SE B	β
Neighborhood socioeconomic status	0.01	0.02	0.10
Police station	0.06	0.05	0.22
Medical clinic	0.00	0.04	−0.01
Hospital	0.02	0.05	0.08
Social Welfare Dept.	−0.01	0.07	−0.02
Homeless shelter	−0.05	0.07	−0.13
Homeless food service	0.06	0.06	0.17
Well lit streets at night	0.01	0.10	0.02
Public parking	−0.02	0.08	−0.04
Public transportation	−0.03	0.08	−0.05
Gas or service station	−0.03	0.04	−0.14
Library	−0.05	0.04	−0.20
Large supermarket	−0.07	0.05	−0.29
Large shopping mall	0.08	0.05	0.25
Mini-market or strip mall	−0.02	0.04	−0.09
Economically depressed feeling	0.03	0.08	0.09
Empty buildings or lots	0.06	0.07	0.13
Streets deserted during the day	0.00	0.04	0.00
Streets deserted during the night	0.05	0.03	0.21
Other buildings are well kept	0.07	0.00	0.16
Streets clean or free of litter	0.06	0.09	0.16
Trees or greenery planted on streets	0.04	0.01	0.11
Homeless persons observed sleeping in neighborhood at night	−0.14	0.08	0.34
Homeless persons seen 'hanging-out' on streets during the day	0.17	0.09	0.48
Pawn shops visible	0.00	0.06	0.01
Intoxicated persons observed on the streets	0.10	0.15	0.37
Drug persons observed on streets	−0.11	0.15	−0.41
Drug dealing observed on streets	0.07	0.05	0.26

$n = 160$ dwellings.

reported little use overall, only 34.5% of OHs maintained complete abstinence over the entire 2-year period. An ANOVA analysis indicated that OHs in the four neighborhood types did not differ with respect to cumulative abstinence rates. A regression analysis examined whether the presence or absence of the reported environmental variables discussed above (i.e., immediate neighborhood amenities and community factors) predicted 12-month house-level cumulative abstinence rates. As shown in Table 3, none of the variables, including neighborhood socioeconomic status, significantly predicted mean slopes of cumulative setting or house-level abstinence from alcohol and drugs.

Power Analyses

Because many of the above analyses supported the null hypothesis, we conducted post hoc power analyses (see Cohen, 1988) to determine if our findings related to a lack of statistical power. For the chi-square analyses, with an n of 160, results indicated fairly large power (.76) to detect "medium" effect sizes ($p < .01$, one-tailed for all analyses). With 160 OHs, medium power existed for the ANOVA analysis (.52) and the regression analysis (.47). These findings suggested the null regression findings were likely not due to lack of statistical power. Supporting the null hypothesis was desirable in this study because it demonstrated that OHs were similar and effective across a range of environmental settings.

DISCUSSION

Within a U.S. national sample of Oxford Houses, we found remarkable similarity regarding interior or exterior dwelling characteristics and operational procedures across different socioeconomic neighborhoods. These results replicated other studies with different, smaller samples of OH residents (e.g., Ferrari, Jason, Davis, Olson, & Alvarez, 2004; Jason et al., 2003) and were consistent with other studies on the ecological impact of recovery dwellings for successful abstinence post treatment (Hitchcock, Stainback, & Roque, 1995; Huselid, Self, & Gutierres, 1991; Smith, Meyers, & Miller, 2001). It seems that a grassroots approach for the expansion of a mutual support program on addiction recovery may effectively meet the personal needs of residents, regardless of community socioeconomic status (Jason et al., 2006).

Our environmental data demonstrated considerable similarity in the local neighborhood amenities near and around our sample of OHs despite their being located in different socioeconomic neighborhoods. OHs were located in communities where residents accessed resources and conveniences facilitated adjustment toward independent and substance-free lifestyles. Together with the dwelling characteristics, an OH may become a "home" for men and women residents looking to develop a sense of community while living in safe and sober physical dwellings (Ferrari, Jason, Olson, Davis, & Alvarez, 2002).

There were several methodological limitations in the present study. For instance, it was not possible to obtain data from every participant in each OH; therefore, we used a conservative method to ensure a sufficient number of participants in each home. It may have been useful to obtain estimates related to other characteristics of the OHs (e.g., housing prices or U.S. census neighborhood data) to confirm the socioeconomic characteristics of the neighborhoods. Future studies might acquire information from all OH members and more economic information about the neighborhoods. We only examined variables within the immediate (i.e., 2-block radius) house environment; future studies might focus on OH settings within a larger ecological framework. Finally, future research assessing neighborhood characteristics of recovery homes should consider a sample of individuals who engage in greater substance use.

Nevertheless, OH residents remained "clean and sober" from alcohol or drugs at the one-year mark despite important neighborhood environmental differences that may promote relapse. Specifically, some settings had easier access to illegal substances and greater environmental temptations that might prompt alcohol or drug use (e.g., OHs located in lower-class urban areas had the highest proportion of intoxicated or drugged persons observed on the streets). It is remarkable that despite neighborhood socioeconomic status or other neighborhood variables, Oxford Houses maintained high cumulative abstinence rates over a 12-month period. These findings strongly suggest that the Oxford House model of recovery effectively maintained abstinence across a variety of environmental settings, whether middle-class, wealthy, or less prosperous.

REFERENCES

Baumer, E. P., & South, S. J. (2001). Community effects on youth sexual activity. *Journal of Marriage & the Family, 63,* 540–554.

Brown, P., Guy, M., & Broad, J. (2005). Individual socio-economic status, community socio-economic status and stroke in New Zealand: A case control study. *Social Science & Medicine, 61,* 1174–1188.

Cohen, J. (1988). *Statistical power analysis for the behavioral sciences* (2nd ed.). Hillsdale, NJ: Lawrence Erlbaum.

Drukker, M., & van Os, J. (2003). Mediators of neighbourhood socioeconomic deprivation and quality of life. *Social Psychiatry and Psychiatric Epidemiology, 38,* 698–706.

Estabrooks, P. A., Lee, R. E., & Gyurcsik, N. C. (2003). Resources for physical activity participation: Does availability and accessibility differ by neighborhood socioeconomic status? *Annals of Behavioral Medicine, 25,* 100–104.

Ferrari, J. R., Jason, L. A., Blake, R., Davis, M. I., & Olson, B. D. (2006). "This is my neighborhood": Comparing United States and Australian Oxford House neighborhoods. *Journal of Prevention & Intervention in the Community, 31,* 41–50.

Ferrari, J. R., Jason, L. A., Davis, M. I., Olson, B. D., & Alvarez, J. (2004). Similarities and differences in governance among residents in drug and/or alcohol misuse: Self vs. staff rules and regulation. *Therapeutic Communities: The International Journal for Therapeutic and Supportive Organizations, 25,* 179–192.

Ferrari, J. R., Jason, L. A., Olson, B. D., Davis, M., & Alvarez, J. (2002). Sense of community among Oxford House residents recovering from substance abuse: Making a house a home. In A. T. Fischer, C. C. Sonn, & B. J. Bishop (Eds.), *Psychological sense of community: Research, applications, and implications* (pp. 109–122). New York: Kluwer/Plenum.

Ferrari, J. R., Jason, L. A., Sasser, K. C., Davis, M. I., & Olson, B. D. (2006). Creating a home to promote recovery: The physical environments of Oxford House. *Journal of Prevention & Intervention in the Community, 31,* 27–40.

Hitchcock, H. C., Stainback, R. D., & Roque, G. M. (1995). Effects of halfway house placement on retention of patients in substance abuse aftercare. *American Journal of Drug and Alcohol Abuse, 21*, 379–390.

Huselid, R. F., Self, E. A., & Gutierres, S. E. (1991). Predictors of successful completion of a halfway–house program for chemically-dependent women. *American Journal of Drug and Alcohol Abuse, 17*, 89–101.

Jason, L. A., Davis, M. I., Ferrari, J. R., & Anderson, E. (2007). The need for substance abuse aftercare: A longitudinal analysis of Oxford House. *Addictive Behaviors, 32*, 803–818.

Jason, L. A., Ferrari, J. R., Davis, M. I., & Olson, B. D. (2006). *Creating communities for addiction recovery: The Oxford House model.* Binghamton, NY: Haworth.

Jason, L. A., Ferrari J. R., Dvorchak, P. A., Groessl, E. J., & Molloy, P. J. (1997). The characteristics of alcoholics in self-help residential treatment settings: A multi-site study of Oxford House. *Alcoholism Treatment Quarterly, 15*, 53–63.

Jason, L. A., Olson, B. D., Ferrari, J. R., & Lo Sasso, A. T. (2006). Communal housing settings enhance substance abuse recovery. *American Journal of Public Health, 91*, 1727–1729.

Jason, L. A., Roberts, K., & Olson, B. D. (2005). Neighborhoods and attitudes toward recovery around self-run recovery homes. *Journal of Community Psychology, 33*, 529–535.

Oxford House, Inc. (1988). *Oxford House manual.* Silver Spring, MD: Oxford House, Inc.

Shohaimi, S., Luben R., Wareham N., Day, N., Bingham, S., Welch, A., et al. (2003). Residential area deprivation predicts smoking habit independently of individual educational level and occupational social class. A cross sectional study in the Norfolk cohort of the European Investigation into Cancer (EPIC-Norfolk). *Journal of Epidemiological Community Health, 57*, 270–276.

Smart, R. G., Adlaf, E. M., & Walsh, G. W. (1995). Neighborhood socio-economic factors in relation to student drug use and programs. *Journal of Child & Adolescent Substance Abuse, 3*, 37–46.

Smith, J. E., Meyers, R. J., & Miller, W. R. (2001). The community reinforcement approach to the treatment of substance use disorders. *The American Journal on Addictions, 10*, 51–59.

Measuring In-Group and Out-Group Helping in Communal Living: Helping and Substance Abuse Recovery

JUDAH J. VIOLA, PhD

Psychology Department, National-Louis University, Chicago, Illinois, USA

JOSEPH R. FERRARI, PhD

DePaul University

MARGARET I. DAVIS, PhD

Dickinson College

LEONARD A. JASON, PhD

DePaul University

With a national U.S. sample of communal-living residents in substance abuse recovery, the tendency to help members both inside and outside their community was examined. Study 1 (n = 670) developed the Communal Living In-Group Helping Scale to distinguish helping directed toward housemates vs. others. Study 2 (n = 419) used this communal helping measure and a general altruism scale to explore gender, ethnicity, and 12-step sponsorship related to in-group (housemates) and out-group (others in the community) behaviors. Results revealed significant sex differences, and significantly higher helping for both men and women was reported among 12-step sponsors along two dimensions. Implications focused on gender-related differences in social helping interactions and in-group formation in recovery communities.

Funding was made possible in part through National Institute on Drug Abuse (NIDA) grants #5F31DA16037 and # R01DA13231. Portions of this project come from the first author's masters thesis under the supervision of the second author and were presented at the 2004 annual meeting of the Midwest Psychological Association.

Numerous research reports indicate several positive long-term psychological and physical health effects associated with helping others (see Brown, Nesse, Vinokur, & Smith, 2003; Smith, Fernengel, Holcroft, Gerald, & Marien, 1994). For example, benefits from helping others include tranquility, improved self-worth, greater optimism, raised self-esteem, as well as decreased depression and helplessness (Luks, 1992). People who frequently engage in helping activities, such as volunteer work or mentoring, experience better perceived physical health and live longer in relation to others who do not perform community service (Andrews, 1990; Moen, Dempster-McClain & Williams, 1992). Helping also affords persons the ability to develop ties and sustain connections with others in their community.

One important application of helping behavior that may have "real-world" relevance is within the field of substance abuse intervention. The effects of the helping processes on the helpers have been rarely studied (Campbell & Campbell, 2000), but the small body of literature that does exist focuses on the topic of persons in recovery providing assistance to peers with similar histories of substance abuse (members of their in-group). Kahn and Fua (1992) found high rates of continued sobriety among people in recovery from substance abuse who served as substance abuse counselors. In learning to be substance abuse counselors, participants gained skills that enabled them to be effective, socially useful, and valued by society and to earn a living by their efforts. Kahn and Fua also reported that participants experienced an increase in self-esteem and self-concept. More recently, Zemore, Kaskutas, and Ammon (2004) reported that helping others by sharing experiences, explaining how to get help, and giving advice on housing and employment emerged along with 12-atep involvement as an important predictor of successful substance abuse recovery. Furthermore, among individuals still drinking at follow-up, helping during treatment predicted a lower probability of binge drinking (Zemore et al., 2004).

However, the motivation and likelihood for helping to occur may differ if the recipients are considered either in-group or out-group members (Gaertner & Dovidio, 2000). *In-group bias*, a well-known phenomenon in social psychology (Schroeder, Penner, Dovidio & Piliavin, 1995; Sherif, Harvey, White, Hood, & Sherif, 1961), was defined by Turner, Brown, and Tajfel (1979) as any instance of favoritism, whether unfair or unjustifiable, in any manner such as perception, behavior, attitude, or preference. In short, in-group favoritism is simply favoring one's own "kind" without substantial reasoning. Researchers have found that persons tend to favor members of their groups in order to foster a social identity (Tajfel & Turner, 1979). Triandis (1994) suggests that establishing group boundaries enables individuals to identify themselves as belonging to either the in-group or out-group and creates security and interdependence among in-group members. In addition, research has shown that in-group members are more likely to be generous, forgiving, and prosocial toward other members of their in-group (Gaertner & Dovidio, 2000).

Research with persons in recovery has not explored the distinction between in-group and out-group helping, or potential sex differences in helping. The distinction between helping behavior in general and helping in recovery may be particularly relevant to the study of recovery processes, given that in-group identification seems to be an integral aspect of recovery (Morgenstern & McCrady, 1993). Early in 12-step substance abuse recovery programs, for instance, individuals are encouraged to personally identify themselves as alcoholics/addicts and seek support and help from members of the group of alcoholics/drug addicts (Alcoholics Anonymous, 1995). The perception that one is accepted by members of an in-group may result in greater optimism about the future, a lessening of the effects of stress, and an increased perceived sense of community (Bishop, Chertok & Jason, 1997; Ferrari, Jason, Olson, Davis, & Alvarez, 2002). Furthermore, persons who feel a part of a group that shares the experience of recovery may display increased levels of empathy and helping behavior (Roberts, Salem, Rappaport, Toro, Luke, & Seidman, 1999).

With regard to helping behavior, in-group–out-group dynamics may affect men and women in different ways. Sex and gender role differences related to helping have been reported in areas such as empathy and prosocial behavior (Skoe, Cumberland, Eisenberg, Hansen, & Perry, 2002; Jaffee & Hyde, 2000). For instance, women typically score higher on self-report indexes of empathy and prosocial personality (e.g., Eisenberg & Fabes, 1998), but men score significantly higher than women on self-reported frequencies of actions (Penner, Fritzsche, Craiger, & Freifeld, 1995). Eagly and Crowly (1986) also reported that in studies of adults' helping behavior in brief encounters with strangers (out-group members), men provided more instrumental acts of helping than women (e.g., carrying heavy packages, helping people with car troubles), and women received more of such help than men. Women compared to men provide more emotional (in-group) support, especially in close relationships (e.g., Zahn-Waxler, Cole, & Barrett, 1991).

One appropriate population with which to develop a measure and then study the links between helping and in-group–out-group affiliation among individuals in recovery may be Oxford House. Oxford Houses (OH) are self-supported, self-governed, communal-living recovery houses for men and women recovering from alcohol and drug addiction without professional staff involvement (Oxford House, 1998). Each same-sex setting utilizes a community-based, social support approach to abstinence from drugs and alcohol where the residents monitor each other's abstinence recovery. At present, over 1,200 Oxford Houses in the U.S., Canada, and Australia are located in middle-class neighborhoods as rented, single-family dwellings that residents of each house self-govern (see Ferrari, Jason, Sasser, Davis, & Olson, 2006). OH residents share the experience of addiction to substances and related hardships (e.g., stigma, housing, family, and other problems associated with substance abuse), share the goal of maintaining abstinence, and spend numerous hours a week resolving conflicts, doing chores, bookkeeping, and interviewing potential residents.

Oxford Houses have been compared with therapeutic communities and found to be similar in their aims (Ferrari et al., 2004). However, OH residents were found to have more personal freedom and self-governance. While neither setting allows for self-destructive behaviors by residents, OH does permit residents personal liberties that are agreed upon by housemates in the form of house rules, whereas therapeutic communities do not allow residents to make their own rules (Ferrari et al.). A recent randomized trial exploring the effectiveness of OH found that participants assigned to a communal-living Oxford House compared to usual care condition had significantly less substance use and criminal involvement, and significantly better employment outcomes after 2 years. These findings suggest that there are significant public policy benefits for these types of lower cost, residential, nonmedical, community-based care options for individuals with substance abuse problems (Jason, Olson, & Ferrari, 2006). Previous research on sense of community suggests that OH residents experience strong in-group cohesion (Bishop, Jason, Ferrari, & Huang, 1998; Ferrari et al., 2002). The shared experiences of OH members are likely to increase reciprocal responsibility and in-group identification.

While all Oxford House members are encouraged to engage in a reciprocal helping process with in-group members, a subpopulation of house members who are also 12-step sponsors may provide even more help than the typical resident. In their role as sponsor they are expected to provide social support for their "sponsee" to abstain from substance use. Huselid, Self, & Gutierres (1991) reported that the amount and helpfulness of support from an Alcoholics Anonymous sponsor predicted successful completion of a halfway-house recovery program for women. Sponsors may benefit themselves as well. The *helper therapy* principle originated by Riessman (1965) asserts that the act of helping others who face similar struggles may have therapeutic outcomes for the person offering the assistance (Wallston, Katahn, & Please, 1983). A key element of this principle is that individuals within a group have a shared experience and identify with others who have suffered in similar ways (Riessman, 1965). Acting as a sponsor might facilitate the learning of important interpersonal competencies. This learning process may lead helpers to experience greater feelings of independence and social usefulness, an increased sense of control, and more willingness to receive help (Riessman, 1990).

Despite the important applied implications of studying in-group helping among persons recovering from substance abuse, there exists no published measure of in-group–out-group helping with men and women in recovery. Although a reliable and valid personality measure of helping behavior in general, the self-report altruism scale (SRAS; Rushton, Chrisjohn, & Fekken, 1981), taps helping directed at strangers and acquaintances (out-group members), there are no similar measures for in-group helping among persons in recovery from substance abuse or any mutual-support network. In Study 1 we developed a new in-group helping scale for residential mutual-help groups. In Study 2 we utilized this new measure as well as the SRAS to assess helping among men and women in recovery from substance abuse to further understand in-group as well as out-group helping among communal-living group members. This second study examined potential differences between men and women as well as sponsors versus nonsponsors who are OH residents.

STUDY 1

Study 1 focused on the development of a new self-report inventory, called the Communal Living In-Group Helping Scale, a 10-item measure designed specifically for persons residing in communal-living settings for recovery, such as OH. The scale ascertained the frequency and types of helping behaviors expressed by communal-living group residents. The 10 new items are not reworded items from the SRAS; instead, the new items were written in the same style and with the same parameters as the SRAS. Because the SRAS does not address helping toward in-group members (i.e., housemates/OH members) it is not specific enough to explore in-group helping among and between people in recovery. After constructing and piloting this new scale, we conducted a factor analysis on the items to determine the psychometric properties including internal consistency and factor structure.

Method

PARTICIPANTS

After the researchers completed the appropriate training in ethical treatment of human subjects and the completed the university institutional review board processes, participants were recruited through a larger National Institute on Drug Abuse (NIDA) funded study of Oxford Houses from across the United States clustered in Washington and Oregon, Texas, Illinois, Pennsylvania and New Jersey, and North Carolina (see Jason, Ferrari, Davis, & Olson, 2006). Only participants who had lived in OH for at least 4 months were included in the present study ($Mdn = 11$ months; $range = 4$ to 125 months). Previous research found that these same-sex dwellings (private, single family homes) housed about 7 employed adults who may or not seek professional help to sustain abstinence, and that residents usually stay for around

12 months before living independently away from their OH setting (Jason et al. provides an overview and assessment of the OH model of recovery).

A total of 670 residents (representing 194 different U.S. Oxford Houses) fully completed the surveys. The sample was composed of 451 men ($M =$ 39.40 years old; $SD = 9.6$) and 219 women ($M = 36.10$ years old; $SD =$ 8.8), ranging from 18 to 67 years of age, which is reflective of the over-all national gender and age composition of OH members, with two men's houses for every women's house (Oxford House, personal communication, September, 1999). Fifty-nine percent of the participants were European American, 33% were African American, 4% were Latino and 4% were of other ethnic backgrounds (similar to the population of Oxford House mem-bers across the country). On average, participants reported slightly over 12 years ($M = 12.43$, $SD = 2.98$) of education (high school diploma or GED), had been paid for work for approximately 15 ($M = 15.3$, $SD = 11.04$) days during the last month, and almost 1 out of every 3 participants ($M = 0.32$, $SD = 0.71$) had one or more dependents to sustain financially. Participants reported an average length of daily poly-substance use (i.e., alcohol and drugs) for nearly a dozen years ($M = 11.85$ years, $SD = 10.42$); a history of criminal charges, such as shoplifting or vandalism (47%) and assault (22%); and spending over a month of time incarcerated prior to entering an OH (65%). These characteristics are representative of the profile of most U.S. residents living in an OH (see Jason, Ferrari, Dvorchak, Groessl, & Malloy, 1997).

SCALE DEVELOPMENT

The Communal Living In-Group Helping Scale was developed as a supple-ment to the self-report altruism scale (SRAS; Rushton, Crisjohn & Fekken, 1981), a valid and reliable uni-dimensional measure of helping behaviors directed toward strangers and acquaintances. Similar to the SRAS, the Com-munal Living In-Group Helping Scale asked participants to rate on a 5-point scale (from 1 = *never*; to 5 = *very often*) the frequency with which they engaged in various helping behaviors. However, the SRAS does not tap into helping directed toward in-group members (e.g., close friends, family, or others in recovery). We created new items meant to supplement the SRAS and increase the relevance of the scale to in-group residents by including questions concerning helping behaviors directed at housemates. The Com-munal Living In-Group Helping Scale includes questions on specific-goal related helping (i.e., helping housemates remain abstinent from drugs or alcohol) as well as questions about receiving help from housemates to tap into the reciprocal nature of in-group helping behavior. In addition, the new measure is unique in that it includes questions concerning individuals' per-ceptions of the influence that their communal-living setting may have had on their participation in helping behaviors.

In order to create the SRAS supplement, the authors initially constructed a pool of 25 items. A team of 15 OH researchers then evaluated the items. According to their suggestions five items were eliminated and several wording changes were made to the remaining 20 items. Next, in accordance with Jason, Fennell, Klein, Fricano, and Halpert (1999), each of the 20 items was rated by persons experienced working with the population of interest. Eight OH alumni (4 adult men, 4 adult women) scored each item on a 5-point scale (1 = *definitely do not agree*, 5 = *very strongly agree*) in terms of how this item is "understandable," this item is "relevant to Oxford House residents," and this item will not be "misinterpreted." The 10 items that received the highest ratings as the most understandable and relevant to OH members and least likely to be misinterpreted were selected for inclusion in this measure. Wording changes occurred as needed and were returned to the raters for input concerning the clarity of revisions.

Sample items for this new measure included, "I have helped a new fellow housemate to get settled at the house and learn the tasks involved" and "I have helped members of the house to get around [bus/taxi fare, ride in car]." A reliability analysis to measure the internal consistency of the 10 items developed for the present study revealed a Cronbach's alpha of 0.83 ($M = 31.76$, $SD = 6.93$; scale range = 10 to 50). See Appendix A for the full version of the Communal Living In-Group Helping Scale.

PROCEDURE

Participant recruitment for the national study included letters and phone calls to house presidents and house visits by members of the study's research team. Additional participants were recruited at the Oxford House national convention. After completing his or her surveys, each participant received a $15 check as a token of appreciation for participating. The surveys utilized for this study were pilot tested and took from 40 to 90 minutes to complete.

Results

Preliminary analyses revealed no significant difference among demographic items (i.e., age, sex, ethnicity, income, level of education, length of residence at Oxford House, alcohol use, drug use) based on the recruitment method. The demographic profiles of participants, described in the section on participants above, were consistent with those reported in previous studies (see Ferrari et al., 2002; Davis & Jason, 2005).

An exploratory factor analysis of the Communal Living In-Group Helping Scale was conducted. Maximum likelihood analysis revealed a three-factor solution with eigenvalues greater than one, explaining 64% of the common variance. A varimax rotation was performed in order to obtain orthogonal

TABLE 1 Varimax-Rotated Factor Loadings of "Oxford House Relevant Helping" Items

Descriptor	Factor 1 "Help-Giving"	Factor 2 "Oxford Influence"	Factor 3 "Abstinence Help"
Settle in and learn	.72		
Calmed	.71		
Transportation	.60		
Obtain needs	.58		
Chores	.41		
Since OH, gave abstinence		.84	
Since OH, more helpful		.65	
Received abstinence			.94
Gave abstinence			.45
Eigenvalues	4.09	1.17	1.06
Percent of variance	40.86	11.66	10.06

Note. n = 459. OH = Oxford House. Values indicate factor loadings > .40.

factor loadings. Table 1 presents the varimax factor structure loadings. A criterion of 0.40 or greater for factor loadings was used: the first factor contained five items (*alpha* = 0.78; *M* score = 15.29; *SD* = 4.12) and was titled *Help Giving,* focusing on whether residents helped other housemates (e.g., "I helped fellow housemates get settled and learn tasks involved.") This factor concerned how often in the previous 6 months a respondent participated in specific helping behaviors as opposed to receiving help. Factor 2 was called *Oxford Influence* and consisted of two items (*alpha* = 0.75; *M* score = 8.31; *SD* = 1.74) and related to participant perceptions regarding how their helping behavior in general has changed because of living in the house, regardless of the target of their helping behavior. (e.g., "Since living in Oxford House I have become a more helpful person in general."). The third factor was labeled *Abstinence Help* and contained two items (*alpha* = 0.76; *M* score = 6.85; *SD* = 2.12) that focused on the reciprocal help to remain abstinent from drugs and alcohol that participants give to, and receive from, their housemates (e.g., "My housemates have actively helped me maintain abstinence/sobriety."). It reflects participant perceptions of how much help they have received from other housemates and how much help they have given to other housemates related to abstinence. One additional item ("My housemates have helped me get a job or pay rent.") did not load highly on any of the three factors (load = 0.26) and, therefore, was excluded from further analyses. Furthermore, while these three factors were significantly intercorrelated, none of the coefficients suggest they are measuring the same construct (*r* = .23–.53, *p* < .01). This outcome suggests an initial index on the validity of separate aspects related to mutual support group helping behaviors. It also should be noted that we conducted an additional factor analysis separately for men and for women. The factor structures that emerged were the same across gender.

Discussion

Study 1 was a first step in establishing reasonable psychometric properties of the Communal Living In-Group Helping Scale. In Study 1, we determined that the scale tapped into three discreet types of participants' perceived in-group helping rates; namely, Help Giving, helping as a result of Oxford Influence, and reciprocal Abstinence Help. The three factors in this scale were subsequently used to explore how the Oxford House environment may differentially affect the helping behavior and recovery process of individuals who choose to move into an Oxford House, looking for a safe, supportive home to maintain their abstinence from drugs and alcohol. Furthermore, since Oxford Houses tend to be run similarly to other communal-living recovery settings (e.g., therapeutic Communities, see Ferrari et al., 2004) the Communal Living In-Group Helping Scale may be a useful tool for examining in-group helping in various recovery home settings. One limitation of Study 1 is that it did not include a test–retest sequence, and thus test–retest reliability is not yet available for this scale. Future research with this scale ought to explore the reliability of the measure over time. Furthermore, Study 1 does not provide information concerning convergent or divergent validity.

STUDY 2

Recent research with OH residents suggests that social support plays a different role in women's recovery than it does in men's (see Davis & Jason, 2005). These findings underscore a need to explore factors that may unfold during and differentially impact the process of recovery for women and men. As noted earlier, some research suggests that among the general population women tend to provide more help than men do to their close friends or family. Furthermore women tend to help more in environments where they feel safe, whereas men tend to provide more help in public and more help directed toward strangers than do women (Eagly & Crowley, 1986; Zahn-Waxler et al. 1991).

Because African Americans often report less satisfaction with substance abuse interventions (Wells, Klap, Koike, & Sherbourne, 2001) and have lower rates of retention in substance abuse treatment (Mertens & Weisner, 2000), it is also important to explore whether there are differences in in-group helping rates between ethnic groups. However, there is no prior published research suggesting differences in helping rates between European Americans and African Americans. Therefore, in our second study we examined ethnic differences between European and African American OH residents on out-group helping (using the SRAS) and in-group helping (measured by factors of the communal in-group helping scale). Study 2 also tested for differences in helping tendencies toward in-group and out-group members between participants who were versus were not 12-step sponsors. Research has indicated that sponsorship in mutual-help affiliations may lead to better outcomes and build skills among sponsors (Huselid, Self, & Gutierres, 1991; Crape, Latkin & Knowlton, 2002).

Therefore, Study 2 utilized the newly developed Communal Living In-Group Helping Scale to explore potential gender, ethnicity, and 12-step sponsorship differences in helping behaviors among OH residents. In order to explore the relationship between gender and helping behaviors, participant scores from the three factors of the Communal Living In-Group Helping Scale as well as a measure of out-group help (SRAS) were collected. Based upon the recent literature suggesting sex differences in recovery and context-dependent helping (Davis & Jason, 2005; Skoe et al., 2002) we predicted that women would report significantly higher scores on the Communal Living In-Group Helping Scale, whereas men would report significantly higher scores on our measure of out-group directed helping (as determined by the SRAS). We predicted that sponsors would report higher rates of helping than non-sponsors across each of the dependent variables, while we explored ethnic difference and helping behaviors related to in- and out-groups.

Methods

PARTICIPANTS

Study 2 included a subset of participants from Study 1. Out of 670 residents included in our first study, only 459 individuals completed both surveys for Study 2 and had similar history of poly-substance abuse (i.e., had abused both alcohol and at least one other drug) to be included. Also, 40 additional participants were excluded from Study 2 based upon their ethnic background because of the very small sample sizes per group (i.e., Native American [$n = 2$], Asian/Pacific Islander [$n = 4$], Latino/a [$n = 22$], "other" [$n = 12$]). Consequently, the second study included 419 persons who identified themselves as either African American ($n = 159$) or Caucasian ($n = 260$) and who self-reported a history of both alcohol and drug abuse. The sample included 291 men (181 Caucasian, 110 African American: $M = 39.94$ years old, $SD = 9.1$) and 128 women (79 Caucasian, 49 African American: $M = 36.75$ years old, $SD = 8.8$). Similar to Study 1, these participants reported an average of 12 years of education (high school diploma or GED), had been paid for work for approximately 15 days during the last month, and more than a third of the sample had dependents to sustain financially ($M = 0.38$, $SD = 0.86$).

PSYCHOMETRIC MEASURES AND PROCEDURE

Demographic information (age, sex, ethnicity, level of education, income, number of dependents) included items from the fifth edition of the Addiction Severity Index—Lite (ASI; McLellan, Kushner, Metzger, Peters, Smith,

Grissom et al., 1992). Participants also completed the *self-deception enhancement (SDE)* subscale of the Balanced Inventory of Desirable Responding (Paulhus, 1988). This 20-item subscale examined the potential for inadvertently deceptive answers to self-reports of questions regarding helping behavior. Participants rated their agreement with each statement along a 7-point scale (1 = *not true*; 7 = *very true*). Paulhus (1988) reported mean scores ranging from 7.5–7.6 (*SD* = 3.2) and 6.8–7.3 (*SD* = 3.1) for males and females respectively, with good internal consistency (Cronbach's alpha ≥ 0.68) and test–retest correlation over a 5-week period of 0.69. The current samples revealed a somewhat lower means across men (*M* = 5.34, *SD* = 3.14) and women (*M* = 4.85, *SD* = 2.76).

All participants completed the 20-item self-report altruism scale (SRAS; Rushton et al., 1981) along with the Communal Living In-Group Helping Scale (developed in Study 1). Participants rated on a 5-point scale (1 = *never*; 5 = *very often*) the frequency with which they engaged in various helping behaviors. Rushton and colleagues (1981) reported respondents' mean scores ranged from 52.01–57.11, (*SD* range = 8.89–11.70) and that the SRAS was internally consistent, with a Cronbach's alpha of ≥ 0.78. The directions for the SRAS were slightly altered in the current study to ask participants to answer each question in reference to the "last 6 months" rather than their lifetime. P. J. Rushton (personal communication, January, 2002) and R. Johnson (personal communication, January, 2002) agreed that for the present study, it would be appropriate to add a phrase regarding a 6-month time frame. Scores on the SRAS with the new directions retained their internal consistency with the current sample, yielding a Cronbach's alpha of 0.85, but did show lower means across men (*M* = 42.11, *SD* = 10.87) and women (*M* = 40.19, *SD* = 9.96). Participants' scores on the Help Giving, Oxford Influence, and Abstinence Help factors of the Communal Living In-Group Helping Scale from Study 1 were also utilized in the analyses below.

Results

Four *Pearson product-moment correlation coefficients* were obtained to examine the relationship between the helping measures and the SDE scale. Significant positive correlations were found between the scores on the SDE and Oxford Influence Helping scores (*r* = .19, *p* < .01), and between the SDE scores and Help Giving scores (*r* = .12, *p* < .01). Consequently, even though these coefficients were rather low in magnitude, all successive inferential analyses concerning the helping measures included SDE scores as a covariate.

Next, a two-way MANCOVA was employed using a 2 (ethnic race: Caucasian vs. African American) × 2 (gender: men vs. women) design, with the SRAS and three factors of the new communal helping measures as dependent variables and social desirable tendencies as the covariate. The multivariate test showed that SDE was a significant covariate $F(4,411) = 4.66, p < .01$. The between-subjects test revealed no significant effect of SDE on SRAS scores or Abstinence Help scores; however, there was a significant main effect for both Help Giving, $F(4,411) = 6.35, p = .01$, and Oxford Influence, $F(4,411) = 15.64, p < .01$. The MANCOVA omnibus test revealed no significant effects of race on any of the helping measures.

GENDER

Even after accounting for the effect of socially desirable reporting (as measured by the SDE), there was a significant main effect (omnibus) for the helping measures, $F(4, 411) = 8.00, p < .01$. With regards to in-group related helping, female compared to male residents reported that they provided more help to housemates over the past 6 months as assessed on the helping scales (Help Giving), $F(1, 411) = 6.58, p = .01$. Compared to males, female residents reported that OH had more positively influenced them to become helpful people in general and that they had done more to help others maintain their abstinence as a result of OH (Oxford Influence), $F(1, 411) = 11.20, p < .01$. Compared to males, female residents also reported more reciprocal abstinence help occurring in their houses (Abstinence Help), $F(1, 411) = 6.17, p = .01$. In contrast, with respect to out-group related helping, $F(1, 411) = 4.73, p = .03$, men reported greater rates of helping strangers and acquaintances that did not live in OH than women.

SPONSORSHIP

An additional item of interest explored in the present study was whether or not serving as a 12-step program sponsor (e.g., Alcoholics Anonymous or Narcotics Anonymous) had an impact on helping behaviors. A subsample of 85 participants reported being sponsors at the time of the survey. In mutual-help organizations, 12-step sponsors are required to provide support to individuals whom they sponsor. Thus, sponsors may have the skills and knowledge of how to help their housemates remain abstinent, and this behavior may generalize from the individuals whom they sponsor to their housemates. Also, individuals who decide to sponsor others through the recovery process may be more helpful people in general than individuals who do not volunteer to become 12-step sponsors.

A 2 (sponsorship: sponsor vs. nonsponsors) × 2 (gender: men vs. women) MANCOVA omnibus test, controlling for SDE scores, revealed that there was a significant main effect of sponsorship, $F(4, 406) = 3.58, p < .01$. The between-subjects portion of the MANCOVA test revealed that even after accounting for socially desirable responding, there were significant main effects of sponsorship for three of the four measures of helping. As expected,

TABLE 2 Mean Scores on the Self-Report Scale Scores

Report subscales	Male ($n = 291$)	Female ($n = 128$)
Total 20-item SRAS	42.26(10.86)	40.34 (9.99)
Help Giving	14.98 (4.04)	16.20 (4.25)
Oxford Influence	8.12 (1.78)	8.68 (1.59)
Abstinence Help	6.66 (2.06)	7.28 (2.17)

Note. Value in parenthesis is standard deviation.

SRAS scores were significantly higher among sponsors than nonsponsors, F (1, 406) = 7.54, $p < .01$. Help Giving was significantly greater among sponsors than nonsponsors, F (1, 406) = 11.36, $p < .01$ and Oxford Influence scores were also significantly higher among sponsors than nonsponsors, F (1, 406) = 7.35, $p < .01$ (see Table 2)

The between-subjects tests also revealed significant sex-related main effects that replicated the findings previously discussed. Specifically, females compared to males reported higher rates of helping on the three factors of OH-relevant helping measure (i.e., Help-Giving, Oxford Influence, and Abstinence Help), with a reverse effect for the out-group helping measure (i.e., SRAS), in which men reported higher scores than women.

Discussion

Significant sex differences were a major finding for Study 2. More specifically, controlling for the effect of social desirability, women compared to men reported providing more help to housemates over the past 6 months (Help Giving), were more likely to report that they helped others maintain their abstinence as a result of OH (Oxford Influence), and reported engaging in more reciprocal help related to abstinence in their houses (Abstinence Help). In contrast, men reported greater rates than did women of helping strangers and acquaintances who did not live in OH.

TABLE 3 Mean Scores of Helping Measure and Subscales by 12-Step Sponsorship and Participant Sex

| Variable | Independent self-report help-giving influence of abstinence help | | | |
	Altruism	Scale	Oxford	House
12-step sponsors ($n = 85$)	44.69 (11.98)	16.88 (4.50)	8.68 (1.68)	8.71 (2.71)
Men ($n = 61$)	45.33 (12.31)	16.64 (4.15)	8.36 (1.81)	8.45 (2.59)
Women ($n = 24$)	43.08 (11.16)	17.50 (5.35)	9.50 (0.88)	9.38 (2.94)
Not sponsors ($n = 329$)	40.63 (9.89)	14.90 (3.95)	8.17 (1.75)	8.13 (2.29)
Men ($n = 226$)	41.08 (9.96)	14.46 (3.88)	8.04 (1.78)	7.90 (2.18)
Women ($n = 103$)	39.66 (9.69)	15.87 (3.93)	8.48 (1.66)	8.65 (2.43)

Note. Value in parenthesis is standard deviation.

This pattern of women providing more help within the home and carrying out similar amounts or less help outside of the home are consistent with the traditional gender role ascribed within American society (Yoder, 2003). It has been noted that as women's comfort level increases, so does their helpfulness. Eagly and Crowley (1986) report that when women are in safer-feeling environments, existing gender differences in helping rates, even with strangers, virtually disappear. In relation to recovery, women in OH have reported strong appreciation for the safe and supportive environment of Oxford Houses (Dvorchak, Grams, Tate, & Jason, 1995) and have reported psychological sense of community both when they enter the homes and after being there for some time (d'Arlach, Curtis, Ferrari, Olson, & Jason, in press). An increased comfort may account for the greater helping tendency reported by women's Oxford Houses. This sex difference did not emerge for helping strangers or acquaintances outside of the Oxford Houses, consistent with past research that has found that men engage in more helping activities than women when helping a stranger (e.g., Oswald, 2000; Hope, Jackson, & Avis, 1988).

The sex differences that emerged in Study 2 were consistent across the different helping factors. Women reported that they were providing and receiving a variety of help in their Oxford Houses. Study 2 adds to prior research on social support by Davis and Jason (2005); it uses a different sample of OH residents and suggests that a recovery model based on social support may be consistent with traits that are traditionally considered feminine, such as nurturing, sharing, and cooperation. Together, these studies argue for the importance of recognizing the differential processes occurring for women in addiction recovery. While more research in this area is needed prior to developing specific suggestions for promoting clinical support to women in recovery, these findings support practices that increase women's comfort so that they can provide and receive support from their housemates during the recovery process. Consistent mutual helping behaviors in and around their homes may increase the likelihood of more consistent and lasting abstinence from drugs and alcohol for women.

Another interesting finding from Study 2 was the significant impact of 12-step sponsorship on helping. Controlling for socially desirable responding, participants who served as 12-step program sponsors scored significantly higher than nonsponsors on the SRAS, the Help Giving, and the Oxford Influence measures. A plausible explanation for this outcome of the present study may be generalization of helping behavior (Nemeroff & Karoly, 1991). That is, because 12-step sponsors are required to provide support to individuals whom they sponsor, they already have the skills and knowledge of how to help their housemates remain abstinent. These skills and behaviors may generalize from the individuals whom they sponsor to their housemates. An alternative explanation is that individuals who decide to sponsor others through the recovery process may be more helpful people in general than individuals who do not volunteer to become 12-step sponsors.

A priori assumptions concerning the physical and psychological health benefits of helping for the helper, based on community and health psychology literature (Brown et al., 2003; Schwartz & Sendor, 2000; Riessman, 1965; Wallston et al., 1983), guided the focus of the present studies toward exploring whether living in OH may serve as catalyst for residents to become more helpful. However, both studies presented here were only a first step toward answering this question. Because of the nature of Study 2's design (i.e., the cross-sectional method), causal statements cannot be made about the effects that emerged over time. Further research using a longitudinal design might be beneficial to understanding changes over time. A repeated measures design also might control potential confounding variables, such as individual differences in altruistic tendencies (e.g., self-concept and self-esteem factors) among OH residents.

GENERAL CONCLUSION

Along with a longitudinal design and additional personality variables that might impact aspects of altruistic tendencies of residents, we suggest that future research attempt to incorporate actual observation of behaviors into the methodology of "real-world" in-group and out-group studies. Together, these methods would triangulate data and attain the most accurate information concerning the frequency of specific helping behaviors.

As more information is gained with regard to building a sense of community and the in-group and out-group influences on helping behavior, female Oxford Houses might be seen as models for recovery homes promoting great potential for success. In addition, consistent with the helper therapy principle, recovery models that encourage individuals to become 12-step sponsors may benefit the recovery of the sponsor as well as the "sponsee" (Crape, Latkin, Laris, and Knowlton, 2002). Therefore, we also suggest that 12-step sponsorship be studied further in its own right for its benefits to the recovery process. Nevertheless, the present studies contribute to a better understanding of altruism and support group processes by developing a brief, reliable, and valid self-report instrument. Furthermore, Studies 1 and 2 add useful information on both helping behaviors in situations of substance abuse addiction recovery and the processes involved in in- and out-groups associated with social support settings.

REFERENCES

Alcoholics Anonymous. (1995). *Alcoholics Anonymous.* (3rd ed.). New York: Alcoholics Anonymous World Services.

Andrews, H. F. (1990). Helping and health: The relationship between volunteer activity and health-related outcomes. *Advances*, 7(1), 25–34.

Bishop, P. D., Chertok, F., & Jason, L. A. (1997). Measuring sense of community: Beyond local boundaries. *Journal of Primary Prevention*, *18*, 193–212.

Bishop, P. D., Jason, L. A., Ferrari, J. R., & Huang, C. F. (1998). A survival analysis of communal living, self-help, addiction recovery participants. *American Journal of Community Psychology*, *26*, 803–821.

Brown, S. L., Nesse, R. M., Vinokur, A. D., & Smith, D. M. (2003). Providing social support may be more beneficial than receiving it: Results from a prospective study of mortality. *Psychological Science*, *14*(4), 320–327.

Campbell, D. E., & Campbell, T. A. (2000). The mentoring relationship: Differing perceptions of benefits. *College Student Journal*, *34*(4), 516–523.

Crape, B. L., Latkin, C. A., Laris, A. S., & Knowlton, A. R. (2002). The effects of sponsorship in 12-step treatment of injection drug users. *Drug & Alcohol Dependence*, *65*(3), 291–301.

d'Arlach, L., Curtis, C. E., Ferrari, J. R., Olson, B. D., & Jason, L. A. (in press). Substance-abusing women and their children: A cost-effective treatment option. *Journal of Social Work Practice in the Addictions*.

Davis, M. I., & Jason, L. A. (2005). Sex differences in social support and self-efficacy for recovering from substance abuse. *American Journal of Community Psychology*, *36*(3/4), 259–274.

Dvorchak, P. A., Grams, G., Tate, L., & Jason, L. A. (1995). Pregnant and postpartum women in recovery: Barriers to treatment and the role of Oxford House in the continuation of care. *Alcoholism Treatment Quarterly*, *13*(3), 97–107.

Eagly, A. H., & Crowley, M. (1986). Gender and helping behavior: A meta analytic review of the social psychology literature. *Psychological Bulletin*, *100*, 283–308.

Eisenberg, N., & Fabes, R. A. (1998). Prosocial development. In W. Damon (Ed.), *Handbook of child psychology* (5th ed., Vol. 3, pp. 701–778). New York: Wiley.

Ferrari, J. R., Jason, L. A., Davis, M. I., Olson, B. D., & Alvarez, J. (2004). Similarities and differences in governance among residents in drug and/or alcohol misuse: Self vs. staff rules and regulations. *Therapeutic Communities: The International Journal for Therapeutic and Supportive Organizations*, *25*, 179–192.

Ferrari, J. R., Jason, L. A., Olson, B. O., Davis, M. I., & Alvarez, J. (2002). Sense of community among Oxford House residents recovering from substance abuse. In A. T. Fisher, C. C. Sonn, & B. J. Bishop (Eds.), *Psychological Sense of community: Research applications and implications*. (pp. 109–122). New York: Klewer/Plenum.

Ferrari, J. R., Jason, L. A., Sasser, K. C., Davis, M. I., & Olson, B. D. (2006). Creating a home to promote recovery: The physical environments of Oxford House. *Journal of Prevention & Intervention in the Community*, *31*, 27–40.

Gaertner, S. L., & Dovidio, J. F. (2000). *Reducing intergroup bias: The common ingroup identity model*. Philadelphia: Psychology Press.

Hope, S. L., Jackson, H. F., & Avis, M. J. (1988). Helping: The effects of sex differences and locus of causality. *British Journal of Social Psychology*, *27*(3), 209–219.

Huselid, R. F., Self, E. A., & Gutierres, S. E. (1991). Predictors of successful completion of a halfway-house program for chemically-dependent women. *American Journal of Drug & Alcohol Abuse*, *17*(1), 89–101.

Jaffee, S., & Hyde, J. S. (2000). Gender differences in moral orientation: A meta-analysis. *Psychological Bulletin, 126*, 703–726.

Jason, L. A., Fennell, P. A., Klein, S., Fricano, G., & Halpert, J. (1999). An investigation of the different phases of the CFS illness. *Journal of Chronic Fatigue Syndrome, 5*(3/4), 35–54.

Jason, L. A., Ferrari, J. R., Davis, M. I., & Olson, B. D. (Eds.). (2006). *Oxford House: A decade of collaboration.* New York: Haworth Press.

Jason, L. A., Ferrari, J. R., Dvorchak, P. A., Groessl, E. J., & Malloy, J. P. (1997). The characteristics of alcoholics in self-help residential treatment settings: A multi-site study of Oxford House. *Alcoholism Treatment Quarterly, 15*, 53–63.

Jason, L. A., Olson, B., & Ferrari, J. R. (2006). An evaluation of communal housing settings for substance abuse recovery. *American Journal of Public Health, 91*, 1727–1729.

Johnson, R. C., Danko, G. P., Darvill, T. J., Bochner, S., Bowers, J. K., Yua-Huang, H., et al. (1989). Cross-cultural assessment of altruism and its correlates. *Personality and Individual Differences, 10*(8), 855–868.

Kahn, M. W., & Fua, C. (1992). Counselor training as a treatment for alcoholism: The helper therapy principle in action. *International Journal of Social Psychiatry, 38*(3), 208–214.

Luks, A. (1992). *The healing power of doing good.* Columbine, NY: Fawcett.

McLellan, A. T., Kushner, H., Metzger, D., Peters, R., Smith, I., Grissom, G., et al. (1992). The fifth edition of the Addiction Severity Index. *Journal of Substance Abuse Treatment, 9*, 199–213.

Mertens, J. R., & Weisner, C. M. (2000). Predictors of substance abuse treatment retention among women and men in an HMO. *Alcoholism: Clinical and Experimental Research, 24*, 1525–1533.

Moen, P., Dempster-McClain, D., & Williams, R. M. (1992). Successful aging: A life-course perspective on women's multiple roles and health. *American Journal of Sociology, 97*(6), 1612–1638.

Morgenstern, J., & McCrady, B. S. (1993). Cognitive processes and change in disease-model treatment. In B. S. McCrady and W. R. Miller (Eds.), *Research on Alcoholics Anonymous: Opportunities and alternatives* (pp. 153–164). New Brunswick, NJ: Rutgers Center of Alcohol Studies.

Nemeroff, C. J., & Karoly, P. (1991). Operant methods. In F. H. Kanfer & A. P. Goldstein (Eds.), *Helping people change: A textbook of methods.* New York: Pergamon Press.

Oxford House. (1998). *Oxford House manual.* Silver Spring, MD: Oxford House.

Oswald, P. A. (2000). Subtle sex bias in empathy and helping behavior. *Psychological Reports, 87*(2), 545–551.

Paulhus, D. L. (1988). Assessing self deception and impression management in self reports: The balanced inventory of desirable responding (Manual available from the author at the Department of Psychology, University of British Columbia, Vancouver, Canada V6T 1Y7).

Penner, L. A., Fritzsche, B. A., Craiger, J. P., & Freifeld, T. R. (1995). Measuring the prosocial personality. In J. Butcher & C. D. Spielberger (Eds.), *Advances in personality assessment* (pp. 10, 147–163). Hillsdale, NJ: Erlbaum.

Riessman, F. (1965). The "Helper" Therapy principle. *Social Work, 10,* 27–32.

Riessman, F. (1990). Restructuring help: A human services paradigm for the 1990s. *American Journal of Community Psychology, 18*(2), 221–230.

Roberts, L. J., Salem, D., Rappaport, J., Toro, P. A., Luke, D. A., & Seidman, E. (1999). Giving and receiving help: Interpersonal transactions in mutual-help meetings and psychosocial adjustment of members. *American Journal of Community Psychology, 27*(6), 841–868.

Rushton, P. J., Chrisjohn, R., & Fekken, C. (1981). The altruistic personality and the self-report altruism scale. *Personality and Individual Differences, 12*(4), 293–302.

Schroeder, D. A., Penner, L., Dovidio, J. F., & Piliavin, J. A. (1995). *The psychology of helping and altruism: Problems and puzzles.* New York: McGraw-Hill.

Schwartz, C., & Sendor, M. (2000). Helping others helps oneself: Response shift effects in peer support. In K. Schmaling (Ed.), *Adaptation to changing health: Response shift in quality of life research* (pp. 43–70). Washington, DC: American Psychological Association.

Sherif, M., Harvey, O. J., White, B. J., Hood, W. R., & Sherif, C. W. (1961). *Intergroup conflict and cooperation: The Robbers Cave experiment.* Norman OK: University of Oklahoma Book Exchange.

Skoe, E. A., Cumberland, A., Eisenberg, N., Hansen, K., & Perry, J. (2002). The influences of sex and gender-role identity on moral cognition and prosocial personality traits. *Sex Roles, 46*(9/10), 295–309.

Smith, C., Fernengel, K., Holcroft, C., Gerald, K., & Marien, L. (1994). Meta-analysis of the associations between social support and health outcomes. *Annals of Behavioral Medicine, 16,* 352–362.

Tajfel, H., & Turner, J. C. (1979). An integrative theory of intergroup conflict. In W. G. Austin & S. Worchel (Eds.), *The social psychology of intergroup relations* (pp. 33–47). Monterey, CA: Brooks/Cole.

Triandis, H. C. (1994). *Culture and social behavior.* New York: McGraw-Hill.

Turner, J. C., Brown, R. J., & Tajfel, H. (1979). Social comparison and group interest in in-group favoritism. *European Journal of Social Psychology, 9,* 187–204.

Wallston, M. M., Katahn, M., & Please, J. (1983). The helper therapy principle applied to weight management specialists. *Journal of Community Psychology, 11,* 58–66.

Wells, K., Klap, R., Koike, A., & Sherbourne, C. (2001). Ethnic disparities in unmet need for alcoholism, drug abuse and mental health care. *American Journal of Psychiatry, 158,* 2027–2032.

Yoder, J. D. (2003). *Women and gender: Transforming psychology* (2nd ed.). Upper Saddle River, NJ: Prentice Hall.

Zahn-Waxler, C., Cole, P. M., & Barrett, K. C. (1991). Guilt and empathy: Sex differences and implications for the development of depression. In J. Garber & K. A. Doge (Eds.), *The development of emotion regulation and dysregulation* (pp. 243–272). New York: Cambridge University Press.

Zemore, S. E., Kaskutas, L. A., & Ammon, L. N. (2004). In 12-step groups, helping helps the helper. *Addiction, 99*(8), 1015–1023.

APPENDIX A: THE COMMUNAL LIVING IN-GROUP HELPING SCALE

For the following items please circle the number that fits your experience on the following scale:

1 = NEVER 2 = ONCE 3 = MORE THAN ONCE 4 = OFTEN 5 = VERY OFTEN In the last SIX MONTHS:

1. I have helped a fellow housemate obtain something important that he or she needed (e.g., a job, a place to live, etc.).

    1   2   3   4   5

2. I have helped a new fellow housemate to get settled at the house and learn the tasks involved.

    1   2   3   4   5

3. I have calmed a housemate who was upset or frightened.

    1   2   3   4   5

4. I have helped members of the house to get around (bus/taxi fare, ride in car).

    1   2   3   4   5

5. I have actively helped members of the house maintain their abstinence/sobriety.

    1   2   3   4   5

6. My housemates have actively helped me maintain my abstinence/sobriety.

    1   2   3   4   5

7. My housemates have helped me get a job or pay rent.

    1   2   3   4   5

8. I have done chores that needed doing without being asked even though I did not have to.

    1   2   3   4   5

9. Since living in Oxford House I have become a more helpful person in general.

    1   2   3   4   5

10. Since living in Oxford House I have done more to help others remain sober/abstinent than I did prior to living in Oxford House.

    1   2   3   4   5

Index